Addiction Medicine Specialist

HOLLY L. GEYER, MD

ENDING
THE
CRISIS

Mayo Clinic's Guide to

OPIOID ADDICTION *and*
SAFE OPIOID USE

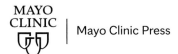

MAYO CLINIC | Mayo Clinic Press

Published by Mayo Clinic Press

The information in this book is true and complete to the best of our knowledge. This book is intended only as an informative guide for those wishing to learn more about health issues. It is not intended to replace, countermand or conflict with advice given to you by your own physician. The ultimate decision concerning your care should be made between you and your doctor. Information in this book is offered with no guarantees. The authors and publisher disclaim all liability in connection with the use of this book.

For bulk sales to employers, member groups and health-related companies, contact Mayo Clinic, 200 First St. SW, Rochester, MN 55905, or email SpecialSalesMayoBooks@mayo.edu.

ISBN 978-1-945564-56-7

Library of Congress Control Number: 2022942504

Printed in the United States of America

When you purchase Mayo Clinic newsletters and books, proceeds are used to further medical education and research at Mayo Clinic. You not only get the answers to your questions on health, you become part of the solution.

To stay informed about Mayo Clinic Press, please subscribe to our free e-newsletter at MCPress.MayoClinic.org or follow us on social media.

Image Credits | All photographs and illustrations are copyright of Mayo Foundation for Medical Education and Research (MFMER) except for the following: p. 19, CREDIT: John Parrot / Stocktrek Images via Getty Images

Some images within this content were created prior to the COVID-19 pandemic and do not demonstrate proper pandemic protocols. Please follow all recommended CDC guidelines for masking and social distancing.

MAYO CLINIC PRESS

Medical Editor
Holly Geyer, M.D.

Publisher
Daniel J. Harke

Editor in Chief
Nina E. Wiener

Managing Editor
Mary M. L. Curtis

Education Specialist
Patricia L. Maus

Art Director
Stewart J. Koski

Production Design
Amanda J. Knapp

Illustration
Joanna R. King, Steven D. Orwoll, Brent R. Staples

Editorial Research Librarians
Anthony J. Cook, Edward (Eddy) S. Morrow Jr.,
Erika A. Riggin, Katherine (Katie) J. Warner,
Morgan T. Wentworth

**Additional contributions from Kirkus Editorial and
Rath Indexing**

Contributors
Jerome Adams, M.D. | Jana Anderson, M.D. | Caroline
Burton, M.D. | Danielle Carlson, A.P.R.N., C.N.S., M.S. |
Casey Clements, M.D. | Sabrina Correa Da Costa, M.D. |
Julie Cunningham, Pharm.D., R.Ph. | Alexandra Curtis |
Kathleen Curtis | Ashley Ebenhoh, R.Ph. | Mark Edwin,
M.D. | Kaylie Evers, M.D. | Halena Gazelka, M.D. |
Margaret Gowan Mester, M.A. | Caleb Haselhuhn, M.A.E.
| Rachel Haring Bartony | Julianne Heathcott, M.D. | Adri-
enne Kaufman, M.D. | Benjamin Lai, M.B., B.Ch., B.A.O. |
Tim Lamer, M.D. | Jenna Lovely, Pharm.D., R.Ph. | Lisa
Marks, M.L.S., AHIP | Tyler Oesterle, M.D., M.P.H. | Debra
K. Oldham, DDS, MAGD | Beverly K. Parker | David
Patchett, D.O. | Ariana Peters, D.O. | Steven Porter, M.D. |
R. Paul Post, M.D. | Christopher Poyorena | Liz Proper,
M.A. | Dominica Rehbein, P.M.P., M.H.A., M.P.H. | Bria
Rice, M.D. | Lynette Scherber | Preston Seaberg, M.D. |
Saul Selby | Jacqueline Stevermer-Bakken | Johnathan
Tom, M.S.N., R.N., CHPN | Priyanka Vijapura, M.D. | Tim
Walsh, M.A., L.P., D.P.A. | Christopher Wie, M.D. |
Terrence Witt, M.D. | Kelly Wu, M.D. | Amy Wulff, M.A. |
Cathy Zehring, R.N.

**A special thank you to Minnesota Adult & Teen
Challenge for their efforts in helping create this book.**

This book is dedicated to those who shared their stories,
those who lost the battle and those who continue
to make a difference.

H.G., P.M. and M.C.

Table of Contents

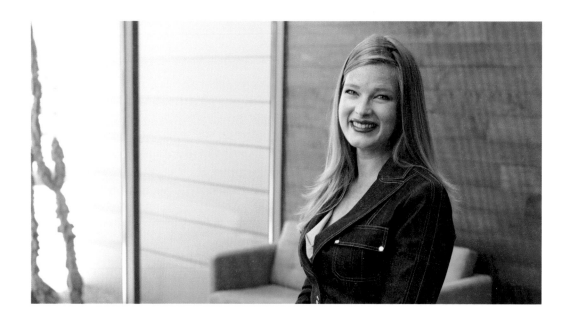

Holly L. Geyer, M.D., is a hospital internal medicine physician and addiction medicine specialist at Mayo Clinic in Phoenix, Ariz. In addition to serving as medical director of Occupational Health, Dr. Geyer leads the Mayo Clinic Arizona Opioid Stewardship Program that works to address safe opioid prescribing and stewardship practices on behalf of the institution. She has served on several Arizona Department of Health subcommittees and is a member of multiple national organizations working to address the opioid epidemic. Dr. Geyer remains actively engaged in research. She lectures nationally on opioid addiction and safe opioid prescribing, and has authored more than 70 peer-reviewed publications, book chapters and educational resources.

To develop this book, Dr. Geyer partnered with two Mayo Clinic colleagues: Mary M. L. Curtis and Patricia L. Maus. Mary has been a managing editor on the Patient Education team in Health Education and Content Services for more than 20 years. She has provided editorial support to the Mayo Clinic Opioid Stewardship Committee since 2017. Mary has experienced the heartbreak of losing someone addicted to opioids. Pat is a registered nurse and wellness coach in the Mayo Clinic Healthy Living Program. As a senior patient education specialist at Mayo Clinic, Pat supported clinical areas including addiction, pain rehabilitation, and the psychiatry and psychology programs. Pat was a member of the Mayo Clinic Clinical Practice Committee Charter Project on Opioid Prescribing Guidelines.

Foreword

There are few things that rival the pain felt from losing someone you love to an opioid overdose. Families often are left wondering whether and how they could have intervened. Were there missed warning signs or opportunities to seek help?

Families might even wonder whether they contributed to their loved one's addiction. Maybe they dismissed mental health issues or failed to dispose of unused prescription opioids that were used for self-medication.

There is one thing that all who have lost someone to an opioid overdose share beyond the pain and sorrow and the "what-ifs" — that is a commitment to wanting to make sure that others don't suffer similar tragedies.

This book is meant to speak to and for all people affected by the opioid epidemic. It's a reminder that despite all the challenges we continue to face in our struggle to prevent, treat and recover from opioid use disorder, we now know more than we ever have about how addiction starts and the steps that can be taken to reduce the chances of substance misuse.

Both harm reduction and medication-assisted treatment — while still underutilized and often not readily available — are becoming much less stigmatized, and recovery-friendly schools, workplaces and communities are becoming more commonplace.

The truth is, while overdose deaths are, unfortunately, more common than ever, so are the tools available to fight them. This book aims to increase opioid awareness and knowledge and provide an answer to every parent, sibling, friend or health care provider who asks, "What should I know about opioids and addiction, and what can I do?"

And to those who have lost a loved one, it's reassuring to know that we are learning more all the time and working toward ensuring that others have a more positive outcome in the future.

Jerome Adams, M.D.
United States Surgeon General, 2017-2021

Why should we care?

1

Why we wrote this book

Opioids. The topic of opioid use and its rise to epidemic proportions has consumed newspaper headlines, nighttime television and social media for decades now.

We've been told to talk to our kids about opioids, ask our doctors about them and intervene on behalf of loved ones misusing them. For some people, opioids have provided a way to regain their lives. But for others, opioids have taken everything.

But what if this book isn't really about opioids?

The word "opioids" is part of the title of this book, so how then could it not be what the book is about? Because the impact of opioids is personal.

At its heart, the book isn't about the drugs themselves — it's about how they impact us and our hope for change. Opioids have affected our health and created pain and uncertainty. They've affected our families, our friends and our neighbors. They've affected our future.

Opioid overdose is now the leading cause of death in adults ages 18 to 45. The influence of opioid overdose is so great that the drugs have even affected American life expectancy — reducing it. These alarming trends have us fearing the worst, and in response, we've begun to view opioids as the enemy. Drugs that we've long trusted to help kill pain are now killing us. As a result, we've grown fearful of what they may do to us when we take them.

BUT WHAT IF . . . ?

What if we choose to fight the myths about opioids instead of the drugs? What would the world look like if we were equipped with information on how to use opioids wisely, store them safely, avoid their risks and reverse their problems?

What if we intervened with loved ones misusing opioids and supported people who seek treatment?

We wrote this book because our world has been fighting the wrong battle. It's time to move our focus away from the battle against opioids and focus, instead, on the real needs of people affected by the drugs.

To each person who reads this book: We've written it to empower you by giving you the tools to prevent opioid-related problems and regain control of your life, health and relationships — or those of a loved one.

People can only fix the problems that they're willing to acknowledge. Solutions require the right information, and we're going to put the most up-to-date knowledge in your hands.

The stories that we share are real stories from real people. They're raw, painful and sometimes disturbing. They're meant to help you understand and remember that problems caused by opioids affect everyday people. Solutions need to come from real problem-solvers.

These stories might be just like your own or people that you know, or they may be different. We invite you to take time to embrace the hopes, fears, regrets and victories of those who may have walked a similar path.

Ultimately, this book isn't about opioids. It's about you.

THREE STORIES

Here are the stories of three people affected by opioids in different ways.

Joyce: "It all goes back to those opioids"

My mother was smart, kind and old-fashioned pretty. She was a good writer, a great cook and a loving grandma. She was a hard worker. She loved John Wayne, snapdragons and elephants. She collected owl pellets and silver spoons. She lived her life serving others. She was grateful for her blessings even though her life was very hard at times. She had a droll sense of humor and an uncanny memory for details. She had plans to be a part of her grandchildren's and great-grandchildren's lives.

And she was addicted to opioids — and the opioids killed her.

Beginning in her late 50s, she had what she would call "a bum knee." Her pain was probably caused by the family legacy of arthritis. All her children tried to get her to have a knee replacement, but she wouldn't do it.

As her pain got worse over the years, she asked her doctors for opioids. And they gave them to her. Lots of them. I guess I knew at the time, but I didn't know enough to realize what a problem this really was. I just thought, "Well, they're helping with her pain, so I shouldn't say or do anything."

I was very wrong.

One spring a few years ago, she was taking more opioids than ever. She got horribly constipated. Then she had a bowel perforation followed by bowel perforation surgery. Then she had complications from the surgery and then she died. In the end, I believe it all goes back to those opioids.

About a month after she died, my brother, sister and I cleaned out her home. I found opioids stashed everywhere: in drawers, in closets, in boxes, even in a jewelry box. I got her medical records and found the notations about all the times she was given a prescription for them. I was horrified no one seemed to keep track of how many she was taking.

I wish I had known a long time ago about the danger of taking opioids. I'm educated. I'm well read. How didn't I know this could happen? I wish I could go back in time and change things. Encourage her to find other ways to manage the knee pain. Go with her to doctors' appointments and advocate for her.

But I can't do those things because it's too late and she's gone. So I'm sharing my story — really her story — with you now.

Pay attention. Speak up. Advocate. Read. Become knowledgeable. Help fight this horrible epidemic. Save someone else's mother.

Penny: "It's my journey too"

My husband and I divorced when our son was a year old. As our son grew up, he and I did lots of things together. We watched movies — he loved the Marvel movies — and we went shopping together. I sat by him as he played video games. We were very, very close. We laughed a lot.

He is articulate. He is smart. He is charismatic. He was an A student at one time. He looks like his dad, but he's got my corny sense of humor.

As a single mom, I did the best I could to keep an eye on him, but I had to leave for work at 6 a.m. He had to get himself up for school and do what he was supposed to.

When he turned 14, I don't know what happened. I figured out he was hanging with the wrong people — kids in local gangs — and that he was addicted to drugs. He got kicked out of school. I would be at work trying to concentrate on my job and I'd wonder what he was doing and what trouble he was getting into.

One day, I came home from work and found a few gang members and some of his bad friends in our home. I kicked them out — and him too. I had to do that, but it was so hard. It was tough love, for me and him. You do these kinds of tough love things — and then you feel guilty.

He went into treatment for his addiction. It took a long time to get him in treatment. Lots of steps and paperwork, but I had to do it. Once he was in, I could catch my breath for at least a few days. That didn't last long.

While he was in treatment, his bad buddies broke into our house, stole our Christmas presents and tazed our dog. It was awful. The dog never recovered and then died. It was all very, very hard, but Steven didn't realize this. Even now, he thinks his addiction is only his problem. I haven't ever been able to get him to see how his addiction affects all of us.

I've had meetings with him and his counselors in treatment. I've really let him have it. I've tried to get him to understand this isn't only about him. One time, I yelled, "You're affecting everything and everyone!" But he doesn't get it. I think he just doesn't see the disaster he creates around him.

There was a time when he was a gifted guitar player. He had electric and acoustic guitars, amps and stands. Even after treatment, he still struggled. I realized his guitar stuff and gaming systems were disappearing. He was selling them to buy drugs.

He's gone into treatment many times over the years. Some programs were inpatient, and some were not. Some were 30-day programs. He lasted in one program for three months.

Long-term programs have worked better for him, but they're expensive and hard to get into. You have to fight with insurance companies. There are usually not enough spaces or housing in programs.

He's gotten into legal trouble. He's stolen a car and set a neighbor's shed on fire. Everything he's done, he's done when he was using. He was with a woman for a while who overdosed and died. He struggled with this a lot. It weighed on his heart. And then he relapsed.

He's 30 now. He lives in and out of halfway houses. He says he's been sober for one year. He's working part-time and has made some progress. It's taken a long time. All the time, though, I wait for more bad news. We do everything we can for him. I don't know what's going to happen when his father and I are gone. I worry about that a lot.

I've had health problems, of course. I've had therapy. I've struggled.

But even after all the problems, he still says, "This is my journey, Mom." I try to tell him it's my journey too.

Charles: "Suffering is suffering"

From NBC News . . . *"This is breaking news about the death of an American music icon. Prince, the innovative, one-of-a-kind artist who's given us so much great music over the decades, has been found dead at his Paisley Park compound in suburban Minneapolis."*

I could not wrap my mind around these words. The world knew the musical icon as Prince, but to me, he was simply my younger cousin.

Prince Rogers Nelson died on April 21, 2016, of an overdose. When I got the news, the room started to spin. None of this made sense, especially when I heard that Prince died of an accidental overdose. Later, the coroner said Prince had ingested pills laced with lethal amounts of fentanyl and similar counterfeit pills were found inside Paisley Park.

As I reflected on my life with Prince, I thought about how we started playing music as little kids. One day, I told Prince we needed a guitar player. He said, "Oh, I can play the guitar." He was 7 or 8 years old and said, "I'm gonna ask my dad for a guitar." A few days later, his father brought the guitar over to my house on Sheridan Avenue North. Prince came back the next day and played "Black Magic Woman" note for note by Santana. I remember looking at him and saying, "I guess you're the guitar player!"

Like many people, Prince suffered from pain. His pain was the result of many years of performing onstage. He didn't have the same options as others to get care for his pain. His every move created news and even salacious rumors. He always tried to make everyone think everything was OK.

My wife and I have met many beautiful people along the way who know the pain of losing a family member to an overdose, and it's so devastating to hear their stories. We were attending a gathering at the Minnesota Capitol Rotunda in St. Paul a few years ago on the opioid bill when a mother approached me and said, "Mr. Smith, I lost my son to an overdose and the pain is unbearable." She genuinely thanked me for having the courage to speak on such an incredible issue.

I've learned through all of this a very important lesson that suffering is suffering, no matter who you are. We need more compassion for people who struggle with addiction. We need to remove the stigma and instead add empathy and support.

———— **WHAT IF** ————

we make an effort to truly understand pain and addiction from the perspectives of those dealing with them? Would our stories have happier endings?

What went wrong? The history of the opioid epidemic

2

If you're reading this book, chances are you've been personally impacted by the opioid epidemic or it's of grave concern to you. Opioids are in the news. They're sold on our street corners. They may be used by someone you love. They may be in your medicine cabinet.

You or a loved one may be intimately familiar with the power of opioids, which are the most commonly prescribed class of pain medication and the number-one contributor to accidental overdose deaths in America.

Since the 1990s, the U.S. has been battling an epidemic of nonmedical opioid use that's claimed nearly half a million lives in overdose deaths. This epidemic has caused immeasurable suffering for innumerable families battling the horrors of addiction.

Between 2020 and 2021, more than 75,000 deaths in the U.S. were attributed to this drug class, and the number of deaths is projected to increase. In addition, the financial toll of opioid addiction in the U.S. exceeds $400 billion per year in health care costs, lost productivity and criminal justice expenses.

With such a broad impact on all elements of daily living, it's no surprise the opioid epidemic has become a top priority within medical and government communities. But to fix the problem, we need to understand how we got here.

In this chapter, we explore the history of the opioid epidemic in America and uncover how misunderstanding of the drugs' power, overprescribing, greed, and lack of regulation have contributed to the drugs' epidemic growth. From its lows to its highs, and everything in between, we'll take a tour through America's opioid history.

PLANTING THE POPPY SEEDS OF THE PROBLEM

For as long as opioids have been available in the U.S., their addictive and destructive potential has been recognized and, at times, exploited. Prior to the 1900s, there was virtually no regulation of the opioid drug class. The importation, distribution and use of the natural opioids morphine and opium poppy were legal without a medical prescription.

Physicians became a driver of the 19th-century opioid epidemic as few options besides opioids existed to manage pain. Many people were advised to take morphine for chronic pain. This resulted in a threefold increase in per capita opioid use between 1870 and 1880.

While early American medical literature contained occasional hints that opioids should be used with caution, few paid much attention to these warnings. Additional concerns about opioids came during the Civil War, when soldiers treated with morphine for injuries developed a lifelong addiction to morphine after the war was over. Many

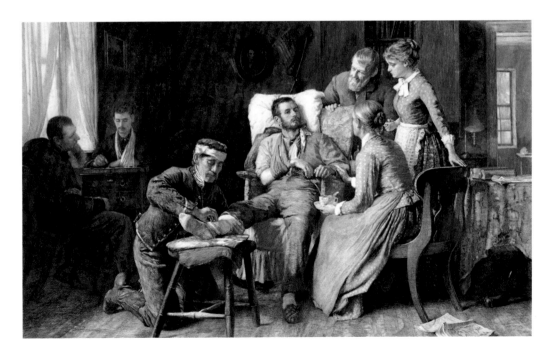

Civil War soldiers were treated with morphine for wartime injuries. Some developed a lifelong addiction to morphine after the war was over.

veterans were so dependent on the drugs, they ultimately overdosed and died.

Similar concerns were noted and vocalized by other countries. In fact, Western countries' illegal importation of opium into China sparked an international war in the mid-1800s.

Complicating the situation was the broad societal belief that overuse of opioids primarily represented a moral deficiency and the stigma that ensued. Suspecting addiction might instead be driven by medical processes in the body, Bayer Pharmaceuticals began distributing another natural opioid in the early 1900s called heroin, which, ironically, was marketed as a treatment for morphine addiction.

The logic behind heroin distribution at the time was similar to today's use of medications for opioid use disorder (MOUD): using one drug to stabilize the cravings for another. (You can read more about MOUD in Chapter 10.) Unfortunately, heroin had its own now-familiar powerful addictive effects, which only fueled the growing problem.

It was time to call in the feds

Crippled by the downstream societal effects of uncontrolled opioid use, many local governments took matters into their own hands in the early 1900s, imposing regulations and restrictions on opioids.

By 1914, the federal government also became involved. The Harrison

WHAT IS OPIOID USE DISORDER (OUD)?

Opioid use disorder (OUD) is the term used for the complex medical condition that results when someone is addicted to opioids. It's one of the most challenging complications of opioid use.

OUD can affect virtually every aspect of someone's ability to function, including personal health, relationships, work and involvement in the community.

You can read more about OUD and how to manage it in Chapter 9.

Narcotics Tax Act was the first federal law to address opioid-related concerns. The act placed a tax on the production, importation and distribution of opioid products within the U.S.

In addition, the act placed the oversight and management of opioids strictly in the hands of prescribers, essentially restricting the drugs' use to pain management. Unfortunately, the act also prevented prescribers from using opioids in ways that could have helped treat addiction. Adding to these efforts was the 1924 Heroin Act, which outlawed all use of heroin.

Through these and other efforts, the U.S. experienced a dramatic decrease in the availability of opioids with a resulting decline in opioid use disorder and overdose deaths. These statistics remained low for the first half of the 20th century.

World War I and World War II served as solemn reminders of the powerful effects of the medications. Returning veterans who were addicted to opioids found themselves reinforcing the broad societal and medical beliefs that the drugs should be used sparingly. By then, physicians were better educated about the serious risks of opioids and limited opioid prescriptions to only certain people, such as those recovering from surgery or an injury.

CHANGING PERSPECTIVES

With the general public and health care providers well aware and wary of complications related to opioids, use of the drugs remained low until the 1970s, when the U.S. began to see a surge in heroin-related overdose deaths. Heroin use spiked dramatically; veterans returning from the Vietnam War found themselves in the grips of opioid addiction as they battled war-related wounds or medicated themselves to treat mental health conditions such as post-traumatic stress disorder.

Health care providers agreed heroin was a detriment to society, but views on prescription opioids began to take on a different focus. Scientific articles began to surface in medical journals suggesting that the risk of addiction to prescription opioids was low, as opposed to the risk of addiction to street drugs such as heroin. Interestingly, drug companies actually wrote some of the more prominent journal articles promoting the use of their brands of prescription opioids.

In 1980, the New England Journal of Medicine published a now-notorious 100-word letter to the journal's editors written by a physician at Boston University Medical Center. The letter addressed the topic of prescription opioids, claiming the painkillers had a low likelihood of causing addiction.

The letter referred to an analysis of 11,882 hospitalized patients, which found that only four patients who received opioids in a hospital showed evidence of addiction. The writer concluded, "Despite widespread use of narcotic drugs in hospitals, the development of addiction is rare in medical patients with no history of addiction."

Several factors combined to create this inaccurate analysis of the data.
- The study limited its focus to only people in the hospital.
- The medical community did not know how to document addiction in patient charts.
- The analysis results were generalized to all people in the hospital without any other supporting information.

This particular article was referenced more than 600 times by pharmaceutical advertising publications, esteemed medical journals and textbooks. The article ultimately laid the groundwork for pharmaceutical companies and health care providers to advocate for opioid use to treat chronic pain not caused by cancer.

It would be the match that sparked a forest fire.

"Stop undertreating pain"

At the same time that opioids were developing an unproven reputation as safe and effective medications for non-cancer chronic pain, several other ideas were gaining traction around pain management. One idea that emerged suggested that health care providers were in general grossly undertreating their patients' pain. Two significant contributors to this idea were the concepts of pseudoaddiction and the introduction of the "Pain as the 5th Vital Sign" campaign.

Pseudoaddiction?

In 1989, the concept of pseudoaddiction was introduced in medical literature. This concept suggested that drug-seeking behaviors of those with a drug addiction were often the same as the behaviors of people with uncontrolled pain. The theory was that the most appropriate therapy for pain was, in fact, more aggressive treatment with opioids.

This idea led to the false assumption that if pain exists, addiction does not. The concept was widely accepted. Because not much was known about the biology that drives chronic pain, the concept was quickly adopted and led to sharp increases in opioid prescribing between 1990 and 2012. In a cruel twist, these prescriptions were written

for many of the people probably most at risk for addiction and overdose.

The push to prescribe for pain

Adding to the situation was increasing pressure placed on health care providers by their patients. Providers who were hesitant to prescribe opioids were soon regarded as uncaring and unsympathetic. Marketing campaigns directed at people in pain encouraged them to ask their doctors for specific opioids.

To better advocate for the patient, prominent organizations led a national health trend introduced as "Pain as the 5th Vital Sign." The campaign's goal was to increase the frequency in which providers assessed and addressed pain. Regulatory agencies then incorporated parts of this campaign into patient assessments.

Every few hours in the hospital setting and during every clinic visit, health care providers asked patients about pain levels and recorded pain scores. Providers were expected to respond to high pain scores just as they would address any other troubling vital sign, such as high blood pressure, an irregular heart rate or an elevated temperature.

Providers regularly asked people about their pain when patients might not have said anything. Even low levels of pain were being treated with opioids in an effort to keep patient satisfaction scores high. This transitioned providers from being opioid gatekeepers to pushing the gates wide open.

When in doubt, follow the money

Government-sponsored regulatory agencies also were paying close attention to the shift in attitudes and the perceived problem of undertreating pain.

Following guidance from the Institute of Medicine (IOM), which published guidelines encouraging a patient-focused approach to medical care, a patient experience survey was created for people to take after being hospitalized. Called the HCAHPS/HCHPS survey, it included questions about pain monitoring and pain control in the hospital. People unwittingly started to use the survey as a substitute for care quality, and survey results soon became linked to national hospital and provider ratings as well as to financial reimbursement to hospitals from the Centers for Medicare and Medicaid Services (CMS).

Given the lean operating budget of most health care institutions, their dependence on government funding, and a goal of wanting to raise patient experience scores, health care providers felt obliged to prescribe opioids when they might not have done so otherwise. Health care providers who felt strongly that opioids weren't in the best interest of the patient often received poor patient experience scores. The low scores potentially impacted their personal pay, career trajectory and self-esteem. This proved particularly frustrating given that multiple studies have refuted the suggestion that patient experience scores accurately reflect quality of care or the chances of having good outcomes.

"Don't worry! Our drug is safer!"

Fully aware of shifting medical views on opioid safety between 1980 and 2000, the pharmaceutical industry both promoted and capitalized on these shifts. It initiated marketing campaigns advocating aggressive treatment of noncancer chronic pain.

By this time, several laboratory-created opioids, such as oxycodone and hydrocodone, had been developed. They were called synthetic or semi-synthetic opioids, and drug companies began to market them as safe alternatives to naturally occurring opioids, even though there was very little data to support these claims. Marketing campaigns by various drug companies were often similarly fraudulent and frequently in violation of federal law.

CHASING PROFIT

Most health care providers, believing opioids were safe and effective tools for

---

WHO WAS HIPPOCRATES?

Hippocrates was a Greek physician who lived from 460 B.C. to 375 B.C. Known for his honor and ethics, he's believed by many to be the father of medicine. The oath physicians take is named after him. The Hippocratic oath is a pledge doctors make to "do no harm."

managing chronic pain, increased their opioid prescribing activities.

The rise of the opioid epidemic was also driven by a minority of providers willing to abandon their commitment to the Hippocratic oath by chasing profit at the expense of patient health and safety. The 1990s and 2000s saw a rapid rise in the number of doctors' offices that provided opioid prescriptions in exchange for cash. These offices were known as pill mills.

In addition, pharmaceutical companies began to hire physicians for speaking engagements who encouraged other physicians to prescribe the drugs — at times, even without medical justification — in exchange for large sums of money. Many drug company relationships were ultimately found to be in violation of anti-kickback statutes and involved outright bribery, resulting in criminal penalties.

WORTHY OF A TITLE: THE OPIOID EPIDEMIC

By 2011, the increase in opioid prescriptions and the problems this was causing

THE U.S. DEPARTMENT OF JUSTICE TAKES ON PURDUE PHARMA

One of the most prominent examples of aggressive and deceptive opioid marketing campaigns was initiated by Purdue Pharma in the 1990s and lasted through the early 2000s. The company began promoting its new long-acting formulation of oxycodone, called OxyContin, for the treatment of chronic pain. Their main audience for this campaign consisted of primary care physicians. Physicians received extraordinary sums of money for prescribing OxyContin and received numerous benefits, including paid vacations.

Purdue Pharma's marketing campaigns promoted OxyContin as being at low risk of causing addiction, even though mounting data suggested the opposite.

In 2020, Purdue Pharma's marketing campaign was ultimately exposed for its criminal activity, including violation of anti-kickback statutes, false advertising and encouraging overprescribing of opioids, resulting in an $8 billion settlement with the U.S. Department of Justice, as well as dissolution of the company.

Other drug companies began facing similar accusations with lawsuits brought by states and cities for charges of "false, misleading and dangerous marketing campaigns" that led to "exponentially increasing rates of addiction and overdose deaths."

had gained national attention. Overdose trends and emerging medical literature made the addictive nature of opioid medications undeniable.

The culmination of misinformation campaigns, failure to regulate prescribing practices and outright greed was enough to kick off the deadliest drug crisis in American history. The Centers for Disease Control and Prevention (CDC) gave the crisis a worthy title: the opioid epidemic.

From 2010 to 2012, average per-person opioid consumption in the U.S. was more than double what it was between 2000 and 2002. At its peak in 2012, overprescribing led to 255 million prescriptions — enough opioids to medicate every American adult with a 5-mg hydrocodone pill every four hours for a month.

America, despite representing only 4% of the world's population at the time, was experiencing up to 27% of the world's drug overdose deaths. By 2015, one-third of American adults were using opioids.

To complicate matters, populations affected by the drug epidemic were changing and expanding. No one appeared to be immune to the potential consequences of these drugs.

From 2013 to 2017, the number of opioid-related overdose deaths nearly doubled from 25,052 to 46,802. From 2009 to 2019, nearly 247,000 people died from prescription opioids. And by 2019, almost 10 million Americans admitted to actively misusing prescription pain relievers.

America had lost control.

The data showed that between 50% and 80% of people dying from opioid overdoses had a history of chronic pain. This made it appear as if most people who were overdosing initially started to take opioids for pain. Yet strangely, prescribing of opioids had started to trend downward around the same time, and prescription opioids were involved in less than one-third of opioid deaths.

So, what was causing these opioid overdoses?

The answer was sobering: The solutions were driving the problem. The reduction in opioid prescriptions that began around 2010 had created a vacuum. People who lacked access to prescription drugs were turning to heroin instead. Heroin overdoses surged nationally from 2010 to 2013 as prescribing of opioids declined.

Unfortunately, the dangers of the illegal drug trade were just beginning. A new class of drugs was on the horizon that would prove more addictive, more available and unquestionably more deadly.

We are referring to the synthetic opioids mentioned earlier in this chapter. Unlike opioids derived from the poppy seed plant, such as heroin and morphine, synthetic opioids were purely lab-created compounds. Some synthetics were closely monitored drugs already used in medicine, such as fentanyl. Others were approved only to be used as tranquilizers for large animals, with no medically approved indication at all. These drugs were strong enough that even two grains the size of a granule of salt were enough to kill a full-grown adult in minutes.

The era of the synthetic opioid crisis took America by storm in 2014. Eventually, more than 25 new synthetic opioids could be purchased as street opioids with little-to-no information on their potency or how the body processed them. Examples included acetylfentanyl, 3-methylfentanyl, sufentanil, carfentanil, thiafentanil, AH-7921, U-47700 and MT-45.

At first, these drugs were mixed with heroin to increase heroin's addictive potential. However, this led to sharp increases in heroin-related overdose rates. Their addictive potential was so powerful that eventually it became apparent that synthetic opioids didn't need to be mixed with heroin. These drugs became the primary illegal opioid product on the market. The resulting trail of damage was unlike anything in American history.

Between 2012 and 2019, overdose deaths skyrocketed due to synthetic opioids, which accounted for 73% of all opioid-related deaths. And the trends continued. Between 2020 and 2021 alone, another 80,000 Americans would lose their lives from problems related to synthetic opioids.

Not only were the drugs inherently more dangerous because of the breathing difficulties they caused, they were also manufactured in unsafe environments. Unlike prescription opioids produced in sterile pharmaceutical environments under the watchful eye of the U.S. Food

and Drug Administration, street drugs were manufactured illegally in home-based labs without any regulatory oversight to monitor for drug purity or contaminants.

People were also taking the drugs in unsafe ways, such as inhaling, snorting and injecting them. These methods greatly increased the risk of overdosing.

In addition, the drugs' effects were more challenging to reverse with standard doses of naloxone, the opioid-overdose reversal agent, and often required multiple treatments to save a life. (You can read more about naloxone in Chapter 6 and Appendix F.) Plus, because many synthetic opioids can't be detected using standard urine drug tests, it was easy for health care providers to miss a medical diagnosis of an opioid overdose.

To make matters worse, illegal opioids were often mixed with other illegal drugs, such as cocaine or methamphetamine, to increase their effects. And the drugs were also frequently contaminated with other nondrug substances, such as talc or flour, to increase the amount of product that could be sold. When injected, these nondrug substances cause serious medical complications.

As the dangers of synthetic opioids became public knowledge, marketing strategies for these street drugs evolved to make the drugs appear safer. Internet sites not readily accessible to the general public, known collectively as the dark web, became a source for pill presses capable of stamping illegal opioids with

THREE WAVES OF THE RISE IN OPIOID OVERDOSE DEATHS

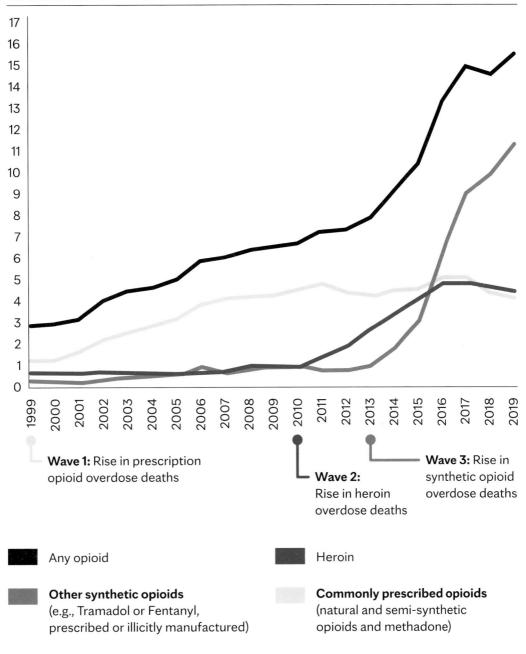

Wave 1: Rise in prescription opioid overdose deaths

Wave 2: Rise in heroin overdose deaths

Wave 3: Rise in synthetic opioid overdose deaths

■ Any opioid

■ Heroin

■ **Other synthetic opioids** (e.g., Tramadol or Fentanyl, prescribed or illicitly manufactured)

■ **Commonly prescribed opioids** (natural and semi-synthetic opioids and methadone)

Source: National Vital Statistics System Mortality File.

titles and numbers identical to prescription opioids. What appeared to be medical-grade pills bought on the street now contained deadly and highly addictive synthetic opioids, such as fentanyl.

The bottom line is that all street drugs were becoming deadlier. And unlike the medical field, in which medications could be regulated with prescribing laws and education, the underworld of street drugs was lawless, ownerless, borderless and increasingly reckless. As a nation, we were beginning to feel powerless.

THE "DUELING 'DEMICS"

In 2017, the U.S. declared the opioid crisis a public health emergency. Opioid-related deaths had doubled between 2010 and 2019, resulting in a decrease in U.S. national life expectancy.

And then along came the COVID-19 pandemic.

Many of the measurable gains in managing the opioid epidemic to that point were effectively reversed. America faced a year of fear, inadequate access to health care, increasing mental health stressors, social isolation and inadequate addiction treatment options. Between 2020 and 2021, these combined issues resulted in a growth in opioid overdoses nationwide — increasing by more than 30% in more than half of the states, with 10 states experiencing a 100% increase.

There were many drivers to these trends. People whose chronic pain had been managed with pain procedures faced closures of their medical clinics. And some people were offered opioids as alternatives to alleviate their pain.

Young people were particularly affected. With shelter-in-place laws and school closures, drug use among adolescents rose dramatically. Drug-related 911 calls increased by 43% for children under age 20, and more than 80% of those calls involved opioids.

Similarly, people struggling with substance abuse disorders were challenged by restricted access to inpatient and outpatient treatment options due to fears of spreading the COVID-19 virus.

Throughout the pandemic, opioid prescription rates remained within expected levels, suggesting street opioids were still the culprit behind growing overdose trends.

However, the U.S. did see some positive changes emerge in 2020 from the COVID-19 pandemic:
• Laws governing the use of telemedicine were loosened, opening doors for people to receive pain management care in rural locations and across state borders.
• Rules about telemedicine for addiction services were also loosened to allow easier access to home-based counseling and provider assessments.

Ultimately, the COVID pandemic highlighted the fragility of current opioid response efforts and set the stage for future management decisions.

MORE THAN BODIES: THE OPIOID TOLL

Few corners of society have escaped the impact of the opioid epidemic. Everyone, whether completing new screenings for opioid-related problems during visits to the doctor or facing an empty chair at the Thanksgiving table, has somehow felt the effects of the crisis.

In addition to the emotional effects, the financial impact of the epidemic has been

BETH : "I SEE SO MUCH NOW"

I've been in law enforcement for six years now, four of those as a county sheriff. Being in law enforcement has been a big eye-opener for me. There's a lot that goes on that people don't realize.

I see how opioids affect families and how the cycle continues. I know of a juvenile female whose mom has been in and out of prison. The daughter is now into prescription drugs. She's going down the same path as her mom.

I see people taking prescription opioids that aren't theirs. I think people have figured out how to work the system. I think some people find ways to get prescriptions for the pills by making doctors believe they need them and then people sell the pills.

I see traffic stops where we find prescription pills in cars and the pills don't belong to anyone in the car.

I see how opioids affect crime in our community. People need money to buy drugs to feed their addiction, so they make bad choices and commit crimes like stealing to get money to buy the drugs.

I see a lot of domestic violence caused by addiction. When people use drugs, they become more violent. Then their children see it. The pattern continues because we know that kids who grow up seeing domestic violence either do it themselves or become victims of it.

I witnessed a paramedic give a man who was overdosing naloxone. When the man came to, he was mad he'd been given naloxone because we took his high away. He was mad we saved his life!

I've seen a child in kindergarten growing up in the substance abuse world. It's already a norm to him at 5 years old. I've seen CPS take kids out of homes whose parents are addicted. I know of a child only a year old who tested positive for substances.

We need more resources: more funding for education and more funding for places to help people with addiction.

I see so much now.

steep. According to the Council of Economic Advisers, between 2015 and 2018, the opioid crisis cost Americans $2.5 trillion. To put this number into perspective, consider that America's annual revenue in 2018 was just shy of $3.5 trillion. Reduced workforce participation, treatment costs and overuse of the U.S. health care system for drug-related medical complications were just some of the factors that contributed to the rising costs.

These trends continue to skyrocket. According to the CDC, the financial impact of opioid misuse and overdose is now estimated to be more than $1 trillion annually.

Health care and criminal justice systems have become strained by the epidemic. Emergency room visits have increased by more than 30% in some areas. Criminal justice costs alone total an estimated $7.7 billion each year, with an estimated 65% of inmates meeting the criteria for addiction.

The inmates' problems don't end at the time of prison discharge: An estimated 75% of those who enter prison addicted to drugs relapse within just three months after release, frequently with a return to

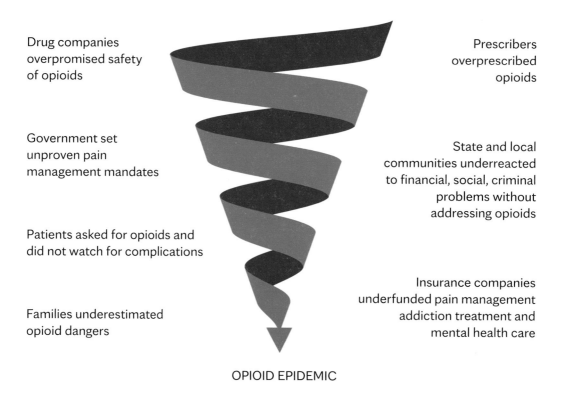

Drug companies overpromised safety of opioids

Prescribers overprescribed opioids

Government set unproven pain management mandates

State and local communities underreacted to financial, social, criminal problems without addressing opioids

Patients asked for opioids and did not watch for complications

Insurance companies underfunded pain management addiction treatment and mental health care

Families underestimated opioid dangers

OPIOID EPIDEMIC

Many factors have contributed to the opioid epidemic spiraling out of control.

criminal behaviors if their addiction isn't addressed.

Society also continues to bear the burden of the epidemic with the breakdown of families. Caregivers addicted to opioids frequently fail to meet role obligations, leaving children caught in the crossfire of addiction and the foster care system.

Recognizing the many factors that have contributed to the epidemic, the U.S. has mounted one of the most robust, multi-organizational interventions in its history — a collective partnership between professional societies, federal agencies, state legislatures, departments of health, medical boards, insurance companies, private corporations, medical communities and people taking opioids or otherwise affected by them — basically, the entire nation.

Some responses were well coordinated and based on changes with a history of success. Other responses were community driven and based on new approaches. All involved were convinced it was time to end this crisis.

The influence of these many interventions has been mixed and, for some, may not be felt for years to come. In the next chapter, we will look at the many ways the U.S. has begun to tackle the opioid crisis and how the efforts worked.

——— **WHAT IF** ———

we stop repeating our mistakes and, instead, start learning from them?

3

America takes on the epidemic

The opioid epidemic. Now it had a name. It was a problem with growing numbers and in clear need of a solution. The next decade would be marked by the most robust national drug crisis response efforts in U.S. history.

Working cooperatively, medical and mental health communities, as well as regulatory and government agencies, developed a comprehensive package of solutions. Many were aimed at curbing overprescribing and mitigating consequences of drug use.

The undertaking would not be without its challenges. Some interventions would revolutionize prescription and substance abuse management industries. Others would prove controversial.

In this chapter, we separate fact from fiction — including the seemingly far-fetched — as we examine efforts to address the opioid epidemic and better manage issues associated with addiction.

WHO CAUSED THE OPIOID EPIDEMIC?

By 2010, initial efforts were already underway to address the epidemic. But addressing it was like putting a puzzle together: You needed all the pieces to create a clear picture. As key players discussed how they were affected, the puzzle quickly grew from a simple 25-piece brainteaser to a 1,000-piece enigma.

Virtually all of society was impacted by opioids. It naturally followed that everyone had a perspective.

Lawmakers were frustrated by the limited regulatory oversight of opioid prescribing and the illegal drug trade on the streets.

Prescribers were frustrated by government funding that rewarded high patient satisfaction scores at the expense of safe prescribing practices. They were also frustrated by the lack of consistent, federally sponsored, evidence-based guidelines for safe prescribing.

Pharmacists were struggling with legal rules requiring them to fill prescriptions they were not comfortable filling.

People lost faith in the government and in health care providers. They became fearful of opioids, convinced one pill could land them in a morgue.

The criminal justice system reached its breaking point as drug-related offenses consumed time, filled beds and stretched budgets.

Communities and families begged for a cure to a problem that had no boundaries.

As a growing number of people brought their concerns forward, everyone wanted the answer to one question: Who was truly responsible for the opioid epidemic?

Over the next decade, the answer became apparent. It was the same answer that generations before knew but failed to accept. For all involved — patients, providers, private insurers, politicians and the public sector — opportunities had come and gone to do better. In other words, everyone was responsible.

Inaction had led to incalculable costs. Everyone needed to speak up, partner up and clean up all things opioid related.

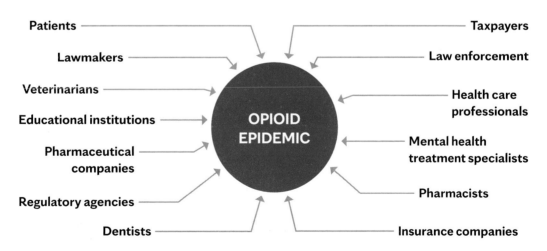

All of society contributed to the opioid epidemic.

GROWING PROBLEMS, FEW SOLUTIONS

Examining the years leading up to 2012 confirmed the truth of this statement: At the end of the day, no one was as guilty as everyone.

Providers had been overprescribing opioids and under-referring to subspecialty services, such as addiction treatment and pain management programs.

Patients had been over-requesting opioids and under-monitoring for complications.

Families had been underestimating the potential of opioids to cause problems and were often little involved in the care of loved ones taking them.

The government had been underfunding opioid crisis efforts and overburdening the health care system with unproven pain management mandates.

Insurance companies had been underfunding pain, mental health and addiction treatment coverage.

Drug companies had oversold the safety of the medication and often promoted their use in unsafe ways.

States and local communities had under-reacted to the mounting financial, social and criminal problems caused by the crisis without fully addressing the driving source.

Everyone had played a role.

IN THE BEGINNING

Early efforts to deal with the crisis were done without broad collaboration. At the federal level, government leaders tried to increase funding for mental health treatment and to reform insurance reimbursement processes.

In addition, they tried to increase the availability of drug courts and to address the importation of illegal substances from abroad.

Medical societies independently developed practice guidelines to influence safe prescribing practices. Health care providers embarked on research related to opioid prescribing and safety.

Unfortunately, there was minimal reform at the state level, and few states had laws that specifically addressed the management of opioids.

TIME FOR A UNIFIED RESPONSE

By 2016, the U.S. had reached its breaking point. It was time to act. Between 2016 and 2020, America faced the opioid epidemic head-on, engaging in robust national efforts and campaigns to inform, empower, enable, regulate and monitor the key players who were handling opioids.

Here are some of the most important changes that were made to address the opioid epidemic.

Prescription regulation

While the link between opioid overprescribing and its deadly consequences was becoming clear, the definition of "overprescribing" was not. In the absence of standardized descriptions and policies for opioid prescriptions, health care providers were left to determine best practices on their own.

In 2016, the CDC released a federally supported reference document for safe prescribing to treat chronic pain. The tool offered guidance to primary care providers who were prescribing opioids to

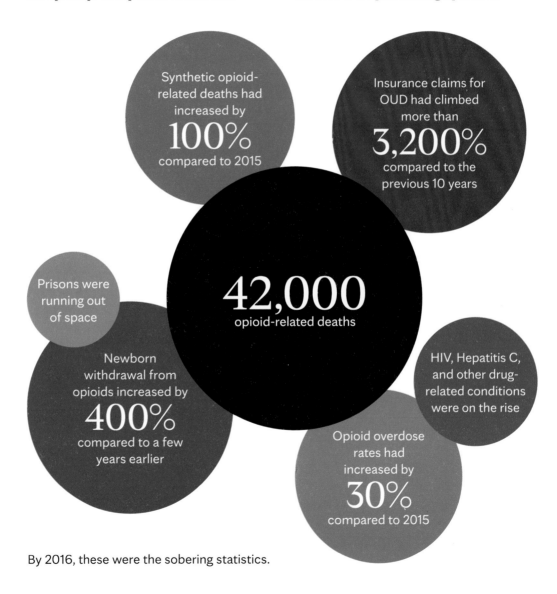

Synthetic opioid-related deaths had increased by **100%** compared to 2015

Insurance claims for OUD had climbed more than **3,200%** compared to the previous 10 years

Prisons were running out of space

42,000 opioid-related deaths

HIV, Hepatitis C, and other drug-related conditions were on the rise

Newborn withdrawal from opioids increased by **400%** compared to a few years earlier

Opioid overdose rates had increased by **30%** compared to 2015

By 2016, these were the sobering statistics.

people with chronic pain. The content came from experts in a variety of medical fields and made recommendations based on the best available evidence.

Guidelines included:
• When and for whom chronic opioid use was reasonable.
• Maximum safe dosing.
• Recommended monitoring of people on chronic opioid treatment.
• Alternatives to opioids for pain management.
• How to address concerns about opioid use disorder.
• How and when to consider discontinuing opioid treatment.

State and local officials struggling with the social and financial burdens of the opioid crisis were desperate for solutions. Guided by the belief that overprescribing was the root of many opioid problems, legislators quickly turned concepts stemming from CDC guidelines into law.

More than 30 states raced to adopt statutes, rules and regulations that limited opioid prescribing. Some states incorporated the CDC guidelines appropriately, basing their laws on patient needs. Some states went well beyond the published guidelines, which focused on chronic prescribing, to include limitations on prescribing drugs for acute illness, injury and surgery.

Most laws focused on capping opioid prescriptions by duration or dose. Many also incorporated other CDC guidelines. State medical boards penalized inappropriate opioid prescribing to the point of

threatening prescribers' licenses if they prescribed outside the established limits.

Insurance companies and pharmacies also adopted components of the guidelines, capping doses per prescription, independently of what the health care provider prescribed.

Has this been helpful?

Between 2017 and 2018, there was an impressive 12% reduction in opioid prescriptions in the U.S. Many prescribers embraced the new recommendations with relief. With the ability to base decisions about the dose, type and duration of opioid prescriptions on scientific evidence, they could more readily manage hostile conversations with people who tried to insist on being given an opioid.

Within the first year following publication, the CDC guidelines were often misapplied. For example, the CDC guidelines focused on people 18 and older who had chronic pain. However, in real-world practice, health care providers were inappropriately using these guidelines for people receiving active cancer treatment, sickle cell disease in children and people with acute pain immediately after surgery.

Providers were also stopping opioid treatment without having discussions with patients or even giving warning. Reports soon emerged of suicides and of people buying illegal opioids rather than not having prescribed opioids to manage pain.

The overall impact on reducing prescribing remains controversial.

Screening people before prescribing

Health care providers know that specific factors can greatly increase the risk of opioid-related complications, such as overdose and addiction. Recognizing this, states have increasingly adopted laws mandating screening for these risk factors before prescribing opioids.

Screening has come in the form of:
- Evaluating for organ dysfunction to prevent opioid problems and overdose.
- Screening for the risk of addiction. This may include a mental health assessment and obtaining a family history of mental health problems.
- Performing regular urine drug screening or counting the number of pills remaining in a bottle, called pill counts.

As of 2017, 26 states required risk and screening assessments in some form.

Has this been helpful?

Some people believe that because of increased screening, people are less likely to experience complications from opioids, such as side effects, overdoses and addiction.

Others say they feel stigmatized because of their risk factors, which can become a barrier to receiving necessary medical care.

Using prescription drug monitoring programs (PDMPs)

Prescription drug monitoring programs (PDMPs) are online state-run database systems that typically include lists of controlled substance prescriptions, including opioids, filled by people living in that state.

The purpose of the system is to reduce overprescribing and "doctor shopping." In addition, the databases serve as tools for law enforcement to identify when opioids are taken by people who weren't prescribed the drug. This is called drug diversion.

Typically, only prescribers, public health officials, law enforcement and other investigating agencies can access the databases. As a result of the epidemic, checking these databases is now mandated prior to prescribing a controlled substance, particularly opioids, in most states.

Has this been helpful?

CDC data has correlated the database's use with a decrease in opioid prescriptions and opioid-related deaths. Some states have seen up to a 50% reduction in oxycodone overdose deaths since implementing the program.

But not all studies have shown that using PDMPs affects opioid overdose rates. Additionally, the websites are run by states, and many don't contain data from other states. Some prescribers find the

PDMP websites challenging and time consuming to use.

Patient education and opioid treatment agreements

The importance of educating people about the risks and benefits of opioids was deemed so critical that by 2017, 26 states had adopted legislative mandates requiring informed-consent conversations before providers prescribed opioids.

Not all states have taken the same approach to education. Some require verbal confirmation while others mandate that people complete a written checklist confirming they understand each talking point.

Some states require people to complete and sign an opioid treatment agreement (OTA) to ensure they understand and agree to their responsibilities while taking the drugs.

Has this been helpful?

People can be empowered to make safe decisions when they're educated about the risks and benefits of taking opioids. Use of OTAs helps to not only ensure that people are aware of their responsibilities but also inform other providers about specific prescribing protocols. Most studies, however, haven't proven that OTAs reduce the risk of adverse opioid-related events.

**HARM REDUCTION STRATEGIES:
WHITE FLAGS OF SURRENDER OR LIFESAVERS?**

Harm reduction strategies are part of public health programs aimed at reducing overdose deaths and dangerous behaviors stemming from nonmedical use of opioids and illegal drugs.

Harm reduction involves a range of policies and services, including medications for opioid use disorder (MOUD), needle exchange programs, places to safely inject, fentanyl test strip distribution and deregulation of naloxone.

Critics of harm reduction say the strategies are like surrendering to addiction. However, communities that have tried harm reduction strategies have found they significantly reduce overdose deaths, the spread of infectious diseases and even the nonmedical use of dangerous drugs. In addition, they offer people struggling with substance abuse a way to get treatment that may be easier than other routes.

Requirements for naloxone co-prescribing

Naloxone is a medication that quickly — but only temporarily — reverses an opioid overdose. To date, all U.S. states have passed laws expanding naloxone access. Naloxone has even been made available for pharmacists to dispense without a prescription. (You can read more about naloxone in Chapter 6 and Appendix F.)

Has this been helpful?

Studies have confirmed that improved naloxone access and distribution correlate with reductions in opioid overdose deaths. Through prescriber education and expanded patient access programs, naloxone prescriptions saw an eightfold increase from July 2016 to 2020.

However, laws requiring naloxone to be prescribed any time an opioid is prescribed have typically been only for specific circumstances. This has limited the number of naloxone prescriptions written.

Needle exchange programs

Needle exchange programs, also known as Syringe Service Programs (SSPs), are government or privately run services that allow people using IV drugs to exchange their used needles for clean ones.

Considered a harm reduction strategy, the primary goal is to help prevent consequences of IV drug use, such as viral bloodborne infections. SSPs also serve as a critical intervention point for people who take drugs. They do this by offering other services, such as:
- Naloxone kits.
- Training for drug overdoses.
- Drug treatment referrals.
- Medical evaluations.
- Post-needle exposure medications.
- Other support services.

Data showing the effectiveness of needle distribution in reducing drug-related complications has led to their dramatic expansion over the past 10 years. Endorsed by the CDC and formally incorporated into their opioid epidemic response, SSPs are now operating in 41 states as of 2019.

Has this been helpful?

More than 30 years of research indicate the effectiveness of SSPs in reducing rates of HIV and viral hepatitis. These programs have also shown reduced rates of overdose deaths and increased enrollment in drug treatment programs. As it turns out, SSPs are often the lifeline to substance abuse services. These programs:
- Are safe for people who take drugs and the public.
- Do not promote additional community crime or illegal drug abuse.
- Are cost-effective.

Many people, however, still have strong concerns that the programs promote illegal drug use and a sense of lawlessness within a community.

Fentanyl test strips

Fentanyl test strips are small pieces of paper capable of detecting fentanyl. Their purpose is to alert the person using opioids of potential fentanyl contamination of a drug. They're fairly inexpensive and easy to use and only take minutes to interpret. The test strips are considered a form of harm reduction with the goal of reducing opioid-related overdoses.

Has this been helpful?

Studies suggest some people who take drugs are more likely to change their drug use behaviors when they know about fentanyl contamination. This includes choosing not to use drugs or at least making sure to have naloxone on hand. Test results can also give information about whether a dealer can be trusted to provide fentanyl-free products. Such test strips are often provided at needle exchange sites.

Critics of fentanyl strips have expressed concerns that offering test strips promotes drug use and other risky behaviors associated with it.

Drug courts

Despite having just 5% of the world's total population, the U.S. houses approximately 20% of the world's prisoners. Recent estimates show that up to one-fifth of the incarcerated population (456,000 people) is serving time for a drug charge. Up to 65% of incarcerated people struggle with

addiction. Incarceration of drug offenders is estimated to cost $3.3 billion annually.

Years of research have confirmed that putting people in prison for drug-related offenses doesn't result in decreased drug use or fewer arrests and overdoses. Only 11% of people with substance use disorder ever receive treatment for the condition during incarceration.

As a result, the concept of using drug courts as an alternative to standard criminal justice pathways has become increasingly attractive. Drug courts are specialized court docket programs that help criminal defendants and offenders, juvenile offenders, and parents with pending child welfare cases who have alcohol and other drug dependency problems.

Drug courts ensure offenders are offered medications for opioid use disorder (MOUD), mental health treatment and counseling services.

Has this been helpful?

People who go through drug courts are less likely to reoffend. They're also less likely to test positive on parole drug screening tests. It's estimated that drug courts save states an average of $5,680 to $6,208 per offender. As of 2020, more than 3,700 drug courts exist in the U.S. in all 50 states and the District of Columbia.

Critics have voiced concerns that drug courts reduce the consequences associated with drug use. Those in the program often serve reduced prison sentences or complete sentences through a court-adjudicated treatment program. Some believe that offenders haven't fully paid their debt to society. Those within the program may also be at risk of stigma for their disorder.

Some also believe that the referral process for drug courts isn't standardized in most settings, with people offered wide variability in treatment.

Increasing access to OUD treatment

Among people with a substance use disorder, people with opioid use disorder are some of the least likely populations to seek treatment. In fact, only an estimated 3.3% of people with OUD pursue outpatient drug treatment services. Lack of insurance coverage, challenges to receiving treatment referrals and the social stigma attached to the disorder have all historically been barriers to treatment.

Passage of the Affordable Care Act (ACA) helped prevent insurance companies from denying coverage or increasing costs of premiums on the basis of preexisting mental illnesses or substance abuse disorders, prevented lifetime limits to services and expanded services to Medicaid populations in addition to those with private insurance.

Initiatives to increase the number of health care providers able to prescribe drug treatment medications became a national priority. Training requirements for prescribing drug treatment medications have been relaxed. In addition, regulations increased the number of people with OUD a prescriber could treat. Many states now require providers to have referral policies for cases of suspected OUD.

Has this been helpful?

People with OUD now have much greater access to treatment through appropriate referrals and better insurance coverage.

Some people believe that not enough has been done to reduce the social stigma associated with OUD. They believe many don't seek treatment due to how it may impact their social stature, employment, relationships and other aspects of life.

A RISING DEATH COUNT DESPITE INTERVENTIONS

Despite the aggressive national interventions described in this chapter, overdose death rates continue to climb. How is this possible?

One explanation may be that reductions in opioid prescriptions have driven people to search for illegal drugs.

An estimated 40% to 86% of current abusers of illegal opioids began their drug use by misusing prescription opioids.

Prescription abuse is rising. In 2001, lifetime nonmedical prescription opioid use (recreational opioid use) was 1.8%. This rate increased to 11.3% in 2013.

However, other data show some states were seeing growing trends in illegal opioid use and overdose deaths long before changes were made to prescribing practices.

One important piece of data remains: Despite significant reductions in opioid prescribing, the U.S. is still the world's leading consumer of opioid prescriptions on an average per-person basis.

GARRETT: "I FELL INSTANTLY IN LOVE"

Growing up, I had a somewhat normal childhood. I played football and lots of other sports. Then I had a football injury and I was prescribed oxycodone.

I fell instantly in love.

That's where my addiction took hold. At 16, I did anything I could to get my hands on more opioids. I began selling other drugs to support my habit. I eventually was raided by the DEA.

Two years later, I started working with a friend who introduced me to fentanyl. I had never heard of fentanyl, but he told me that it was a lot like oxycodone, so I said, "Why not?"

After using it three days in a row, I woke up to opioid withdrawal, something I had never experienced before. I was miserable and I would have done anything to make the misery stop.

Eventually, the fentanyl would no longer cut it and I moved on to IV heroin. It didn't take long before I had my first overdose. I fell in front of a cash register in a gas station and had to be given Narcan. When I woke up, I was scared — but not scared enough to make a permanent change.

After my first overdose, one of my good friends overdosed but unfortunately wasn't as lucky as me. This friend's death led me into a relapse, which caused my second overdose. This time, I had to be given six doses of Narcan to be brought back from the dead. I was dead for 20 minutes and somehow was brought back to life for a second chance.

I went to treatment shortly after this overdose, but I relapsed again. I had another overdose where, luckily, I didn't need Narcan. I blacked out in a gas station bathroom.

I was at my wits' end. This forced me to make the decision to check into treatment. I have just recently celebrated two years of sobriety.

AN EVOLVING PROBLEM

The opioid crisis has wound its way through the entire tapestry of American culture, and because of this, our drug problem has evolved into everyone's problem.

Bit by bit, we continue to come up with solutions, but much more needs to be done. And it can be. Through knowledge sharing and a collective commitment to end this crisis, it is possible to redesign the future.

In the next part of this book, you'll read why and how health care providers use this drug class and how opioids impact pain. You'll learn how to partner with loved ones and providers to limit opioid-related complications and manage them if they arise.

We'll explore the science that drives the controversy and attempt to demystify the risks, benefits and real-world complications of opioids.

——————— W H A T I F ———————

*we propose solutions bigger
than our problems?*

2

All things opioid

FINDING THE WAY OUT

So far, you've read about the tremendous challenges that face our nation when it comes to the opioid epidemic. It's time to talk about a way out, and that's what the rest of this book will do.

To the millions who struggle with pain, we share information about proven tools to help relieve it. If you're offered opioids for treatment, we tell you how to use them safely. If you're currently bound by the chains of addiction, we'll help you create a plan to get free.

To those of you close to a person facing the challenges of opioid use disorder, we empower you to be part of the solution, and we'll show you how you can help.

To the countless health care providers trying to unravel the tangled threads of opioid laws and guidelines, we explain safe opioid prescribing and opioid use disorder (OUD) referrals.

To the lawmakers and social advocates whose voices can bring legitimate community solutions, we provide the big-picture view of the epidemic, and we highlight the tools that can lead to success.

To everyone reading this book, know that you are able to effect change.

As you explore the chapters that follow, ask yourself, "How does my unique experience fit into the opioid crisis? How can I contribute to the solution?"

You'll see a common and sobering theme emerge as you make your way through the content: No one is immune to the effects of the crisis. In one way or another, everyone has felt its biological, psychological, financial, social and spiritual impacts.

The epidemic's worst outcomes are frequently driven by very preventable problems. When providers don't educate patients, people overdose. When people don't follow safe storage instructions, children empty the medicine cabinet. When regulators and lawmakers don't follow the science, pain goes uncontrolled, and people look for other ways to manage it. When families don't know the signs of addiction, treatment is delayed.

And when we choose to do nothing, someone dies.

Don't be afraid to ask questions. Communication and partnership are proven foundations on which to build solutions. The past several decades have shown that breakdowns in communication and partnership have been the key drivers of the crisis. Good communication and partnership can be the key drivers to solving our problems.

Regulators, health care providers and people who take opioids are not the enemy — and neither are the drugs themselves. If we're to move from victims to victory, we need to understand the most basic truth about this drug class: What makes opioids scary is their mismanagement.

When responsibly prescribed, sensibly regulated and offered to the right person for the right reason, in the right form, at the right dose and for the right length of treatment, opioids are one of modern medicine's greatest assets. But dysfunction in any of these processes inevitably contributes to the epidemic.

At the beginning of this book, you read stories from real people who have faced facets of the opioid epidemic. In the pages ahead, you'll read more stories. The themes may be your own. We include them to encourage empathy, education, empowerment and, above all, change.

Right now, perhaps you feel isolated, discouraged or overwhelmed. It's a lot to take in. But understand there's hope and there's help to be found. Join us as we explore the heart of the epidemic and the heartbeats of those who share in its struggles.

——————— **WHAT IF** ———————

*we commit to creating the
future we want?*

Let's talk about opioids

Over the past decade, opioids have become a well-established yet controversial drug class that has commanded the world's attention. We hear about opioids on the news as overdose death rates soar and street versions covertly traffic their way into our communities. We learn from friends that opioids and syringes have been found in their teens' sock drawers.

Maybe we don't fully understand the risks of opioids when medical providers give us a prescription. We stash them in our medicine cabinets anticipating their potential future benefit after our next do-it-yourself construction project.

Opioids are everywhere and they serve a valuable purpose. But at what point do they stop serving us? How does the help that they provide become a problem that can destroy us?

In this chapter, we explore the complex world of opioids. It's important to remember that when taken by the right person, for the right reason, in the right form, at the right dose and for the right length of treatment, opioids can be an effective part of an overall pain management plan.

This book may contain unfamiliar terms. Appendix D is a glossary that includes definitions of many terms related to opioids.

WHAT EXACTLY ARE OPIOIDS?

Opioids are a powerful class of medications meant to be used for a short time after an injury or surgery to manage acute pain and enable activity. Drugs that fall into this class include morphine, oxycodone, hydrocodone, hydromorphone, fentanyl and the illegal drug heroin.

The term "opioid" is often used interchangeably with the term "opiate," but this isn't always correct. **Opiate** refers specifically to naturally occurring drugs that come from the opium poppy plant. Examples of opiates include morphine, codeine and heroin.

Opioid is a more generic term that includes not just opiates but also drugs that were invented in a lab — synthetic and semi-synthetic opioids. Synthetic opioids (fentanyl, methadone) are completely developed through a chemical process. Semi-synthetic opioids (oxycodone, hydrocodone and hydromorphone) have chemical changes made to the original opium plant.

Technically, all opiates are opioids. In this book, all drugs in this class are referred to as opioids. From a government perspective, opioids are controlled substances. This means they're federally regulated and can only be prescribed or administered by people who have a license to do so.

HOW DO OPIOIDS WORK?

When opioids enter a person's bloodstream, they work their way toward nerve cells and attach themselves to opioid receptors. Receptors are anchoring points on the surfaces of cells that combine with specific entities, such as hormones, antibodies or drugs.

When opioids bind to these receptors, they trigger a series of chemical reactions. One of those reactions is to block pain signals, primarily in the central nervous system.

Think of a lock and key. You need a key to fit the lock so you can open something, right? Opioids work much like the key that triggers the lock.

Other effects of opioids

Opioid receptors are also located on cells in other parts of the body, not just those in the central nervous system. When opioids attach to receptors on non-nerve cells, they can cause side effects.

One example of this is in the gastrointestinal (GI) tract. When opioids bind to receptors in the GI tract, they often cause constipation.

Opioids can also bind to certain parts of the brain, causing breathing problems or chemical reactions that lead to addiction. In Chapter 9, you'll read more about how addiction occurs.

WHAT AFFECTS HOW OPIOIDS WORK?

The various types and forms of opioids differ in many ways. Here are the main reasons opioids affect the body differently.

Route

How an opioid is metabolized in the body — or whether it is even metabolized at all — depends on many factors. However, one of the most impactful factors is the route: how a drug enters the body.

Most often, if an opioid is swallowed, it passes through the liver to be metabolized. This can make the opioid less likely to bind to receptors or to do so more slowly. The effects of the opioid are slower.

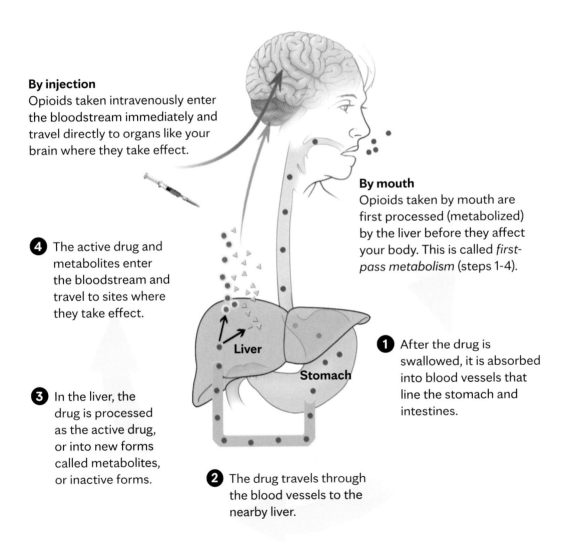

By injection
Opioids taken intravenously enter the bloodstream immediately and travel directly to organs like your brain where they take effect.

By mouth
Opioids taken by mouth are first processed (metabolized) by the liver before they affect your body. This is called *first-pass metabolism* (steps 1-4).

4 The active drug and metabolites enter the bloodstream and travel to sites where they take effect.

1 After the drug is swallowed, it is absorbed into blood vessels that line the stomach and intestines.

Liver

Stomach

3 In the liver, the drug is processed as the active drug, or into new forms called metabolites, or inactive forms.

2 The drug travels through the blood vessels to the nearby liver.

The effect an opioid has on you depends on how it enters the body.

When an opioid is taken by another route, such as intravenously (by IV), it doesn't need to be metabolized to have an effect. Since opioids taken by IV bypass the metabolic process, they bind to receptors more quickly. The drugs go directly into the bloodstream and then into the central nervous system. The effects of the medication are quicker.

For example, morphine given by mouth reaches the receptors more slowly. It takes longer to relieve pain with a pill compared to when it's administered by IV.

Potency

The potency of a drug determines the amount or dose necessary to have an

---

DRUG ROUTES

An opioid can enter the body through many routes. This table shows the medical terms you may hear a provider use to describe the "route" of a medication, which means how you take it.

Route	Definition
Oral	Placed in the mouth and swallowed
Sublingual	Absorbed under the tongue
Buccal	Absorbed between the gums
Intranasal	Absorbed through the nasal passages
Transdermal	Absorbed through the skin
Intramuscular	Injected into the muscle
Implantation	Delivered by a device that has been implanted into the tissue or muscle
Intrathecal	Injected around the spinal cord
Subcutaneous	Absorbed under the skin
Intravenous	Injected into the veins
Rectal	Inserted into the rectum
Inhalation	Inhaled through the mouth or nose and absorbed through the lungs

effect. This means a dose of one type of opioid isn't equivalent to the same dose of another opioid when it comes to providing pain relief or causing side effects.

Opioids with stronger potency are often used for more severe pain. And they also typically have more serious risks, including a higher risk of addiction. Types of opioids with high potency include fentanyl, oxycodone, intravenous hydromorphone (Dilaudid) and methadone.

Dose

Like most medications, opioids come in different doses. These are often measured in milligrams (mg) or micrograms (mcg). No matter what type of opioid is used or how it enters the body, usually, higher doses of opioids are more likely to lead to better pain control. But higher doses also lead to increased risk of side effects, overdose and death.

Because of differences in potency, the dosage of one type of opioid isn't inter-

ROBIN: "WAY OUT OF CONTROL"

I'm 39 years old and I used opioids for 10 years. I began to take them for chronic pain from fibromyalgia and Ehlers Danlos Syndrome. My doctor prescribed five Percocet a day for me for the pain. I took it for four years. One doctor was prescribing it all that time.

It didn't take long before I wasn't swallowing it, but instead, snorting it. Then I started snorting double the amount to get the same effect. It got way out of control! The pills would run out before I was due to refill my prescription. Then I would get withdrawal symptoms, which were horrible.

I wish to God that I had never put that first pill up my nose. It's so bad to do that. Do not do this! I believe snorting

caused the addiction. It was the beginning of the end for me.

I have two kids. It was all about pills when I was raising them. Child Protective Services took my kids. They're with my mom and they're OK now, but the Percocet abuse was part of destroying my family.

When I ran out, I would buy Percocet off the street when I had money. That messed up my finances because I was trying to feed my habit. This led me to use other drugs. Everything was just so bad.

I tell my doctors I struggle with addiction; I tell them to not give me anything. Be sure to tell doctors if you have a history of addiction.

I want a way out.

changeable with the same dosage of another type of opioid. For example, 2 mg of intravenous morphine a day may provide low-risk pain management, but 2 mg a day of intravenous fentanyl can be deadly.

Frequency

"Frequency" refers to how often the drug is taken or administered. Opioids differ in how frequently they need to be taken to maintain an effect within the body. Changing the route of the same opioid can affect how often it should be taken.

For instance, IV fentanyl may be given every two to three hours for pain relief. However, a transdermal fentanyl patch only needs to be changed every 72 hours.

How frequently an opioid is given depends on several factors, such as:
- The route.
- How it is metabolized.
- How quickly the drug is eliminated from the body.

Long-acting opioids

Some opioids are created as extended-release (ER) medications. Other terms for

---

KIDNEY AND LIVER DISEASES AND OPIOIDS

Like all drugs, opioids don't stay in the body forever. Eventually, they're inactivated, eliminated or both.
- "Inactivated" means they're turned into a form that your body doesn't use.
- "Eliminated" means they're removed from your body through its normal waste processes.

Inactivation and elimination often depend on how well the kidneys and liver function. Disease and aging can reduce the ability of these organs to eliminate medications from someone's system.

Kidney and liver function naturally decline as people grow older. This increases the risk of medications such as opioids building up to levels that can cause problems. Problems caused by medications that build up include sleepiness and breathing difficulties.

People who are older or who have kidney or liver disease are often started on a lower dose of an opioid. If they need increased dosages, they are monitored closely.

these are sustained-release (SR) opioids or long-acting opioids. They stay in the bloodstream at a steady concentration for longer periods of time when taken by mouth. Other forms have been developed to be placed on the skin or underneath the skin.

Extended-release morphine (MS Contin) and oxycodone (OxyContin) are common examples. These drugs are usually prescribed only for people who have ongoing pain that isn't expected to diminish with healing, such as cancer pain.

The benefit of a long-acting opioid is that it can reduce the chance of pain spikes, which can happen when shorter-acting opioids wear off. However, long-acting opioids have increased risk of complications and abuse. For this reason, they're not usually prescribed for short-term pain. Long-acting drugs also are given using specific routes, such as by mouth or applied to the skin.

Taking an opioid via a route that isn't approved — such as by IV when the drug is only approved to be swallowed whole — can be deadly.

Short-acting opioids

Opioids that are classified as immediate release only stay in the bloodstream for short periods. They're called short-acting opioids and are often used for short-term treatment of moderate to severe pain, such as after an injury or a surgery.

The more common prescription opioids taken by mouth for moderate to severe short-term pain include oxycodone,

hydrocodone, morphine and tramadol. These are typically taken as needed every four to six hours.

Length of use

Opioids are generally classified for either acute or chronic use.
- **"Acute use"** refers to short-term use, typically a few hours or days.
- **"Chronic use"** refers to taking opioids more than 45 to 90 days on a near-daily basis.

This distinction between these two types of use is very important. This is because studies have shown that the longer someone takes an opioid for acute pain, the higher the risk that opioid use becomes chronic.

Tolerance

The longer a drug stays in your body, the more your body adapts to it. This is done through a process called tolerance. Tolerance occurs as the body gets used to taking a substance, requiring higher doses to have the same effects.

Consider caffeine as an example of how tolerance works:

Susan drinks a lot of caffeinated coffee every day. The coffee doesn't make her jittery because she has a tolerance for caffeine.

John rarely drinks caffeinated coffee, but one day, he drinks a strong espresso full of caffeine. Afterward, he feels jittery and notices a slight hand tremor. This is because he has a low tolerance for caffeine.

Susan decides to stop drinking caffeinated coffee. However, one week later, she breaks down and has a large cup of coffee. An hour later, she notices that she feels jittery and shaky. Susan has lost some tolerance, so the smaller dose of caffeine affects her more.

It takes time, usually weeks, to develop opioid tolerance. People who stop taking opioids even for a week can lose tolerance. This can put them at very high risk for life-threatening adverse effects if they start taking the same dose they were previously taking.

Tolerance becomes an important factor to consider when health care providers change the type of opioid a person is taking. Not only do providers have to calculate the correct dose of the new opioid, but they also have to consider that the person may have a lower tolerance to the new drug.

The right way to change from taking one opioid to another isn't an exact science.

LENGTH OF OPIOID PRESCRIPTION VS. RISK OF LONG-TERM USE

A study done by the CDC showed:

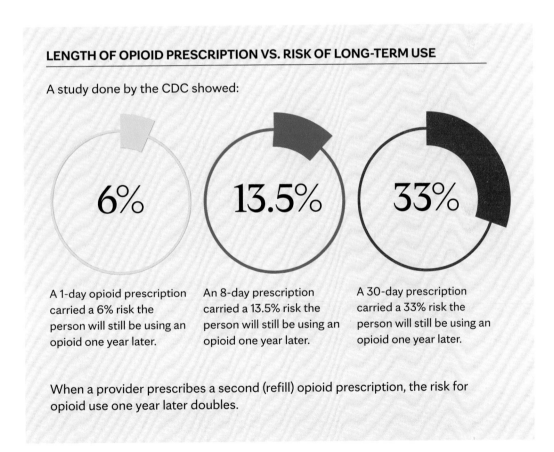

6%

13.5%

33%

A 1-day opioid prescription carried a 6% risk the person will still be using an opioid one year later.

An 8-day prescription carried a 13.5% risk the person will still be using an opioid one year later.

A 30-day prescription carried a 33% risk the person will still be using an opioid one year later.

When a provider prescribes a second (refill) opioid prescription, the risk for opioid use one year later doubles.

Differences between types of opioids as well as other factors can complicate the process.

OPIOIDS: PRESCRIBED AND ILLEGAL

Opioids fall into two main groups:
- Prescribed opioids.
- Illegal opioids, also called street drugs or illicit drugs.

Prescribed opioids

Prescribed opioids come in many forms and differ in their potency. On page 55, you'll find a list of commonly prescribed opioids and the conditions they treat or the reasons they're usually prescribed.

To understand the information provided in the table, keep these things in mind:
- Health care providers usually compare the strength of opioids to the strength of morphine as a way to standardize how strong an opioid is.
- When an opioid is prescribed for acute pain, it's usually prescribed as a tablet or capsule that you swallow. In the hospital or emergency room or during surgery, opioids may be given through a catheter inserted in a vein, called an IV.
- When an opioid is prescribed for chronic pain, some providers choose to use a different route, such as a skin patch or implantable pain pump. Intravenous and intramuscular forms are usually reserved for use in a hospital.

Illegal opioids

Opioids taken without a prescription are called illegal, illicit or street drugs. In this book we mainly address prescription opioids, but it's important to understand

WHAT'S AN ORAL MORPHINE EQUIVALENT?

An oral morphine equivalent (OME) is used to simplify the conversion process when changing the dose a person takes of one opioid to the recommended dose of a different opioid.

The OME chart helps keep the process simple and consistent. Providers use a value on a chart to do the conversion. You may hear your provider use the terms "oral morphine equivalent" or "morphine milligram equivalent."

To switch opioids safely, providers usually need to reduce the dose of the new opioid by 50% from the equivalent dose of the original opioid. The opioid dose can then be increased to achieve pain relief.

PRESCRIBED OPIOIDS

Drug name (generic)	Route	Length of effect	Strength compared to morphine	Common uses
Mild acute pain				
Codeine	Typically swallowed	4 to 6 hours	⅓ as strong	Cough, injuries, pain after surgery
Tramadol	Typically swallowed	4 to 6 hours	¼ as strong	Injuries, pain after surgery
Moderate to severe acute pain				
Morphine	Typically swallowed	4 to 6 hours	—	Injuries, pain after surgery
Hydromorphone	Typically swallowed	4 to 6 hours	4 times stronger	Injuries, pain after surgery
Hydrocodone	Typically swallowed	4 to 6 hours	Same strength	Injuries, pain after surgery
Oxycodone	Typically swallowed	4 to 6 hours	1½ times stronger	Injuries, pain after surgery
Chronic pain				
Buprenorphine	Under the tongue or via a skin patch	Depends on the route	Depends on the route	Chronic pain, treatment of opioid use disorder
Methadone	Typically swallowed	Up to 72 hours	3 times stronger	Chronic pain, cancer pain, treatment of opioid use disorder
Morphine ER (MS Contin)	Typically swallowed	8 to 12 hours	—	Chronic pain, cancer pain
Oxycodone ER (OxyContin)	Typically swallowed	8 to 12 hours	1½ times stronger	Chronic pain, cancer pain
Fentanyl	Patch	Up to 72 hours	50 to 100 times stronger	Chronic pain, cancer pain

that street drugs are much more dangerous than medications given by prescription.

Unlike opioids created in a licensed medical setting, street drugs are produced illegally in nonmedical settings. Street drug use is the leading cause of drug overdose in the U.S.

Street drugs frequently include very powerful and dangerous opioids. Some street drugs are made from the same opioids used in medical settings. Examples are fentanyl and oxycodone. Other street opioids, such as heroin, aren't legal under any condition.

There are tremendous risks involved with taking street opioids. This is primarily because:
- The drugs are often produced in unsanitary environments.
- They're frequently contaminated with other drugs.
- They may contain byproducts that are more powerful and dangerous than the original drug.
- They may contain other nonopioid substances, such as talc, which can be very dangerous.
- There's no government regulation of their potency or dose.
- The drugs are frequently taken using dangerous routes, such as snorting, inhaling or injecting. These routes can increase overdose risks as well as increase the risk of infections or other serious health problems.

Street drugs have been a powerful fuel for the opioid epidemic. Their production in non-pharmaceutical environments, some-

BE CAUTIOUS WHAT YOU BUY

The internet has made it easier to buy many things, including medications. Always be very careful if you choose to buy medications or natural supplements of any kind from websites or someone other than your health care provider.

This is especially true for products being sold as "natural alternatives." There have been instances of people who thought they were buying natural products but instead were sold deadly drugs, including fentanyl.

Talk to your health care provider before using any medication you buy from someone on the internet to ensure the product's use has been well reviewed and validated.

One time, I bought a Percocet that had fentanyl in it. I didn't know that. It was a tiny, tiny pill. My vision got weird, I got really hot and I stopped breathing. I had a seizure too. My family said it happened really fast.

CHEYENNE,
25 YEARS OLD

times called clandestine labs, often results in the purposeful or accidental creation of deadly opioid look-alikes that are up to 10,000 times stronger than morphine.

A look-alike of fentanyl is called carfentanil. Exposure to a dose of carfentanil the size of a grain of salt can be enough to kill a large adult.

Street opioids can also include prescribed opioids taken from medicine cabinets or other locations.

Recognizing that many people trust pills stamped with logos, the makers of street opioids have begun stamping them with similar logos. This makes it almost impossible to distinguish them from legitimately produced opioids.

A more concerning trend has been the contamination of nonopioid street drugs, like marijuana (cannabis), benzodiazepines (lorazepam or Ativan), cocaine and methamphetamine, with opioids.

This contamination makes the nonopioid drug more addictive. The result has been many overdose deaths from drugs that have historically been regarded as safer than opioids.

Safe and effective when used properly

If your health care provider is going to prescribe opioids for you, have an honest conversation about it. Be sure that you understand why you're taking an opioid and how to take it. Then follow your provider's directions very carefully.

In Chapter 5, we examine how health care providers use the information discussed in this chapter to decide whether to prescribe an opioid, which opioid, and for how long. We also examine the side effects of opioids and how to stay safe while using them.

——————— **WHAT IF** ———————

we understand opioids are not always the answer?

5

Using prescribed opioids safely

Given all the negative aspects of opioids, you may wonder why they're still prescribed. Here's why: Opioids — when taken by the right person, for the right reason, in the right form, at the right dose and for the right length of time — are one of our most powerful tools against many types of pain.

However, finding a balance between the benefits of pain relief and the dangers of opioid use can sometimes be challenging. While everyone is at risk for opioid-related problems, some people are at higher risk than others. This, along with other reasons, is often why providers may seem reluctant to prescribe opioids.

Only a small number of medications have or will ever receive the amount of attention given to opioids. Because they're the

deadliest drug class in the medical world, it makes sense to closely examine who should take them and how they should be taken.

In this chapter, we look at the side effects of opioids, as well as safety strategies that can be used to prevent complications. We also discuss how providers carefully balance opioid benefits and risks to determine whether, when and how to prescribe them.

> When taken according to safety guidelines, opioid side effects are usually manageable and rarely life-threatening.

We'll help you understand the value of working closely with your health care provider if you're taking opioids.

Opioids may be controlled substances, but they don't need to control us. Here's how we can stay in control.

GETTING IT RIGHT

Opioids can be a great tool for relieving pain when used by the right person, for the right reason, in the right form, at the right dose and for the right length of treatment. But that's a lot to keep

track of, right? Let's look closer at each of these qualifiers.

The right person

Screening people for potential risks related to an activity in which they are going to take part is a process that can help keep them safe.

Getting ready to depart on an airline flight is one example. A security person has reviewed your ID, scanned your ticket, studied X-rays of your carry-on bag and sent you through a metal detector. These safety practices reduce the risk of harmful acts that might be committed while at the airport or in flight.

When it comes to opioids, health care providers use their own thorough screening process to help keep people safe from opioid complications. Screening before prescribing isn't just recommended: It's the standard of care.

OPIOID PRESCRIPTION CONSIDERATIONS

Health care providers make complex decisions when it comes to prescribing opioids. They consider:

- What health conditions are most appropriate to treat with opioids?
- How should people be screened before they are given opioids?
- When should opioids be started and stopped?
- What complications are possible?
- Who is most at risk for opioid complications?
- How should people be educated on opioid safety, including safe storage and disposal?

WHAT IS "STANDARD OF CARE"?

"Standard of care" refers to treatment that is accepted by medical experts as a proper treatment for a certain disease or condition and that is widely used by health care professionals. This is also called best practice, standard medical care and standard therapy.

If you're going to be prescribed an opioid, you can expect to be screened. If you're not screened, ask your provider about screening for potential opioid complications. There are many factors that can put a person at higher risk of complications. These include:

- Age. People between ages 18 and 45 are at higher risk for opioid use disorder. People 65 and older are at higher risk for overdosing.
- A history of substance abuse.
- Mental health conditions, such as depression or anxiety.
- Unstable home or social circumstances.
- Use of other addictive or sedating medications, such as benzodiazepines or muscle relaxants.
- Breathing issues or heart conditions.
- Kidney or liver conditions.

Some providers use validated screening questions similar to those on the Opioid Risk Tool (ORT) questionnaire.

SAFE OPIOID USE IN CHILDREN AND TEENS

Opioids can be a helpful tool to manage moderate to severe acute pain in children and teens, just as they can be for adults. When used correctly, opioids can help kids do the things needed to help them heal.

However, children and teens are at an even higher risk of complications from opioids. Right now, prescription opioids cause more than half of all opioid overdoses in children and teens younger than 18.

Health care providers most often prescribe opioids to children and teens after surgery and dental procedures. But for many procedures, such as tonsillectomies and teeth removal, ibuprofen has proven effective for managing pain.

Opioid misuse has serious and potentially long-term consequences for children and teens. Because the brain is still developing in young people, children and teens are at high risk of developing opioid use disorder when taking opioids.

Not surprisingly, children who report misusing opioids are 10 times more likely to use heroin as adults than children who didn't misuse opioids as children. Even appropriate use of prescribed opioids before age 18 has resulted in a 33% increase in the risk of opioid misuse later in life.

Storing opioids so that children of any age are unable to access them is essential. Studies show that more than 70% of teens taking prescribed opioids have unsupervised access

The ORT includes questions a health care provider may ask before prescribing opioids to assess the risk of complications.

Having risk factors doesn't necessarily mean that a person can't take an opioid. It just means the provider needs to carefully consider the risks versus the benefits of prescribing opioids to that person, the type and dose of opioid, and the length of time the opioid will be prescribed.

The right reason

Opioids are typically prescribed when someone has:
- Acute pain after an injury or a surgery.
- Tried over-the-counter medications and behavioral pain management techniques that were not effective in managing pain.
- Tried other prescription pain medications that haven't worked.
- Cancer-related pain or another serious

to them. One study found that teens were able to identify where adults were storing opioids even when adults thought they were hiding them.

Unsafe storage and disposal of opioids increase the risk of children and teens using them in inappropriate ways and for nonmedical reasons. They also increase the risk of the medication being taken by someone for whom the drugs were not prescribed, which is both dangerous and illegal.

If you're the parent or guardian of a child or teen who is being prescribed opioids:
- Talk with your child's health care provider about the pain management plan after your child's surgery or procedure. This can help you know what to expect and prevent overuse of medications.
- Ask your child's health care provider about side effects your child may have from opioids and what you can do to manage them.
- Ask about options other than opioids. These may include medications you can buy without a prescription, and nonmedication options, such as ice and heat, movement and other therapies.
- Store opioids in a safe, locked location and dispose of them right away when the drugs are no longer being taken.

Then follow all the safety guidelines for taking opioids explained in this chapter for the best chance of keeping everyone safe.

illness for which there is no expectation of healing or recovery.

There's no conclusive research to support using opioids for:
- Pain originating from damage or dysfunction of the nervous system, such as diabetic neuropathy.
- Chronic pain.
- Pain with no clear source of ongoing tissue injury.
- Pain that continues beyond the expected time frame for healing.
- Pain rooted in psychological conditions, such as depression.

pain and palliative care pain. They may also be an option for people who've developed some tolerance to opioids due to regular use of opioids.
- Intravenous (IV) and intramuscular (IM) opioids may be prescribed for people who are in a hospital or having a procedure and can't take medications by mouth.
- The FDA has approved certain opioids for use only in certain situations, which is another factor in making the decision. For example, certain forms of fentanyl should only be prescribed for cancer pain or end-of-life pain.

The right form

"Form" refers to how the medication is designed to be released into the body. When it comes to choosing the right form of opioid, there are many aspects to consider: Low potency? High potency? Short acting? Long acting? Tablets? Dissolving capsules? Patches? Intravenous? The list of options can seem endless.

The decision about which form to use by which route is usually based on a person's unique needs and medical conditions.

Here is the approach most health care providers take:
- Low- to medium-potency opioids are taken by mouth as needed for acute pain. Examples are tramadol, morphine, hydrocodone and oxycodone.
- Long-acting opioids and opioids in skin patch form, such as oxycodone ER or morphine SR and fentanyl, are used for certain chronic pain situations, cancer

The right dose

Many opioids come in a variety of doses. The higher the dose, the greater the pain

WARNING!

If you take a drug in a manner that wasn't prescribed, this can put dangerously high levels of it into your bloodstream and increase the risk of overdose. Examples of this include crushing a tablet you're supposed to swallow and then snorting it. Even chewing a tablet you're supposed to swallow whole can cause an overdose.

Remember that you should only take opioid drugs in the manner prescribed.

relief, but also the higher the risk of complications, such as breathing problems and overdose.

Health care providers usually start people on a low dose and only move to a higher dose if needed. If someone has been taking an opioid for a long time and the decision is made to change the type of opioid, the provider usually reduces the dose of the new drug by up to 50% to prevent problems, such as an overdose.

To ensure you take the safest dose:
- Don't increase or decrease a dose without first talking with your health care provider. Even small changes in dosage can have a dangerous effect.
- Take the medication at the prescribed time interval. For example, if you're told to take it every 4 hours, don't take it sooner than that. This increases the dose and can be life-threatening.

The right length of treatment

Health care providers should prescribe opioids for the shortest time needed to manage the pain. They often stop prescribing opioids as soon as other medications and other forms of treatment are helpful. Research has shown the following about treatment length:
- The longer length of time someone takes an opioid, the higher the risks of overdose and addiction.
- By limiting the quantity prescribed, the risk of having opioids in the household and available to other people is lowered.
- Overprescribing opioids for acute pain has contributed to an increased supply of opioids in communities. This is directly linked to the upward trend in addiction and overdose.
- The longer the length of treatment, the greater the effects on a person's cardiovascular, gastrointestinal, respiratory, endocrine, immune and central nervous systems. Studies show that long-term opioid use greatly affects these systems, causing more side effects and increasing the risk of serious complications.

It's a complex decision

As you can see, the decision-making process about what type of opioid to prescribe, which route, which form and for what length of time is complex. Influential factors include a person's medical conditions and history and personal situation. Often, it's not a simple decision, and there's no one-size-fits-all answer.

Recent scientific advances now permit gene testing to determine how opioids are processed differently by different people. Companies specializing in this technology provide those who are enrolled with a list of drugs they're most likely to tolerate well and which ones to avoid. The companies are using the science of pharmacogenomics to do this testing. You can read more about pharmacogenomics in Appendix B.

SIDE EFFECTS 101

The point of taking any medication is to have it work for you more than it works against you.

OPIOID SIDE EFFECTS

Side effect	Frequency*	Possible treatments to discuss with your health care provider
Constipation	Very common	Taking a daily laxative, such as: • Sennosides, often called senna • Polyethylene glycol (Miralax) • Lactulose • Magnesium sulfate • Methylnaltrexone • Naloxegol • Naldemedine
Feeling very sleepy	Very common	Taking a lower dose or stopping the opioid altogether. No longer taking medications that cause sleepiness.
Upset stomach and throwing up	Common	Taking the opioid with food or taking a different opioid.
Sleep apnea	Common	Taking a lower dose or stopping the opioid altogether. No longer taking medications that cause sleepiness.
Low oxygen levels	Common	Taking a lower dose or stopping the opioid altogether. No longer taking medications that cause sleepiness.
Depression	Common	Taking an antidepressant or no longer taking the opioid.
Itching	Common	Taking a different opioid.
Inability to urinate, also called urinary retention	Common	Taking a lower dose or stopping the opioid altogether.
Long-term abdominal pain (also known as narcotic bowel syndrome)	Uncommon	No longer taking the opioid.

Side effect	Frequency*	Possible treatments to discuss with your health care provider
Irregular heart rhythm, called arrhythmias (most common with methadone)	—	Ask your health care provider or a pharmacist to closely review for drug interactions that may increase rhythm disorders.
Heart attack/heart failure	—	Taking a lower dose or stopping the opioid altogether.
Dizziness	—	Taking a lower dose or stopping the opioid altogether.
Confusion	—	Taking a lower dose or stopping the opioid altogether.
Increasing pain called hyperalgesia	—	Taking a lower dose or stopping the opioid altogether.
Sexual dysfunction	—	Taking a lower dose or stopping the opioid altogether.
Infertility	—	Taking a lower dose or stopping the opioid altogether.
Low testosterone	—	Taking testosterone replacement therapy.
Osteoporosis and bone fractures	—	Taking bisphosphonates, calcium or vitamin D.
Menstrual cycle changes	—	Taking a lower dose or stopping the opioid altogether.
Breast milk safety	—	Taking a lower dose or stopping the opioid altogether.
Weakened immune system, called immuno-suppression	—	Taking a lower dose or stopping the opioid altogether.

* No consistent research data is available for conditions that have a dash in the frequency column.

The problem with opioids is that this balance can be surprisingly hard to achieve for some people. Opioids are as well recognized for their dangerous and debilitating side effects as they are for their pain-relieving abilities.

The table on pages 64 and 65 lists known side effects from opioid use. Some side effects are more common than others. Some are hard to treat. Fortunately, not all people who take prescription opioids experience side effects.

Higher doses of opioids and more frequent usage generally increase the risk of side effects. For some people, side effects are more noticeable when they first start to take an opioid. For others, the side effects get worse the longer they take them.

Opioids also can interact with other medications known to cause similar side effects and make the side effects worse.

While not considered a side effect, some opioids cause people to feel euphoric.

HEIDI: "IT'S ON YOU"

My husband had knee surgery. Afterward, they prescribed him an opioid.

After we got home, he couldn't stay awake. He was very emotional and he was having pain in his extremities. He couldn't eat and couldn't keep anything down. He said he was having hallucination-type dreams. Weird stuff!

He had taken opioids before for medical reasons, but he never had these kinds of problems. He knew something was very wrong. We both knew.

I called his doctor's office. They asked what he was taking and how much was his dose and I told them. There was silence on the phone.

Then I was put on hold for 20 minutes.

They came back on and said he'd been prescribed three times the dosage he should be taking.

It took him a long while to get better, almost three months.

My advice to everyone is to ask questions before you take anything. Question, question, question! Don't assume what you're being given is right. Ask what they are giving you and why they are giving it to you. Speak up if you think something is wrong.

And super important! Ask about the possible side effects so you can watch for them. Don't blindly take medication.

It's on you what you put in your mouth.

Opioid-induced euphoria is the feeling of intense excitement and giddiness that some people call feeling high or getting a rush. People who experience euphoria are much more likely to become addicted to opioids.

Caution is key

Each opioid is unique, and some have distinctive side effects. Before you start taking an opioid, ask your health care provider these questions:

- What side effects might I experience?
- What can I do to manage side effects?
- How will this opioid interact with any other medications I take?
- Do I need a prescription for naloxone in case of an accidental overdose? (Read more about naloxone in Chapter 6 and Appendix F.)
- What side effects should I contact you about and within what amount of time?
- What side effects should my friends and family watch out for as I take this?

Managing the most common side effects

Most people who take opioids for a short amount of time don't have side effects that become serious problems. If you take an opioid, try the following strategies to manage the most common side effects.

Constipation

Your goal is to have a bowel movement at least every two to three days. Consider taking a bowel stimulant, such as senna, every day to achieve this. If you're still not having regular bowel movements despite taking the bowel stimulant, talk with your health care provider about other medications that may help. Don't take stool-bulking products such as fiber because they can make symptoms worse.

Upset stomach

If you get an upset stomach, try taking your opioid with food. If you still have problems, talk to your health care provider about switching to a different opioid. Some opioids are more likely to cause an upset stomach than others.

Itching

For most people, itching isn't caused by an allergy to the medication. Many times, the cause is the activation of receptors in the central nervous system. When this happens, the itching doesn't respond to allergy medications.

> **WARNING!**
>
> Rarely, some people are allergic to an opioid. Signs of an allergic reaction include hives, itching, swelling, wheezing and difficulty breathing. If you have any of these signs, call 911 or have someone drive you to seek emergency care. Do not drive yourself.

For significant itching, ask your health care provider about taking a different opioid. Don't take an antihistamine that makes you sleepy, such as diphenhydramine (Benadryl). Because an opioid can also make you sleepy, you risk becoming overly drowsy. Antihistamines have also been shown to enhance the effects of opioids, increasing the risk for abuse.

PREVENTING SERIOUS COMPLICATIONS

Many people taking opioids don't have complications, but complications can still happen. Possible serious complications include breathing problems, addiction, opioid overdose and death.

If you're being prescribed an opioid, make sure to tell your health care provider about all medications or substances you take, including herbal products or dietary supplements. Let your provider know if you have a personal or family history of an anxiety or mood disorder.

Also, be open with your provider about whether you or a family member has a history of substance use disorder. Even brief use of an opioid may make these conditions worse.

Make sure your provider knows of any other medical conditions you may have, especially conditions related to your heart and lungs. With certain conditions, opioids may not be safe to use.

You can help prevent complications by doing the following:
- Take the opioid exactly as your provider has instructed. Make sure you understand the instructions and ask questions about anything that is unclear to you.
- Don't take other medications or substances that can make you tired or sleepy. These include alcohol, muscle relaxants and benzodiazepines. If you're not sure whether a medication you take is a muscle relaxant or a benzodiazepine, ask a health care provider or a pharmacist.
- Fill all your prescriptions at one pharmacy so the pharmacist can watch for possible drug interactions.
- Keep naloxone available. Educate friends and family about how to use it. Read more about how naloxone can save a life in Chapter 6. Step-by-step directions about how to administer naloxone are in Appendix F.

WHAT TO EXPECT WHEN PRESCRIBED AN OPIOID

To become educated is to become empowered. A clear understanding of opioids can help people ask questions that keep them and their loved ones safe, watch for problems and determine whether the drugs are having the right effect.

When considering prescribing an opioid for acute or chronic pain, a health care provider may:
- Review the source of pain in detail to determine whether opioids are an appropriate treatment.

- Discuss other pain management treatments.
- Screen for a personal or family history of substance abuse and mental health, heart, lung, kidney and liver conditions.
- Screen for the use of other medications or substances that increase the risk of overdose.
- Review the state prescription drug monitoring program to check whether someone has received opioids, sedatives or other controlled medications in the past. Read more about the PDMP in Chapter 3.
- Discuss the expected benefits for pain and the ability to function, the goals of opioid treatment, the risk of side effects and complications, and safe opioid storage and disposal.
- Prescribe the lowest effective dose in an immediate-release form for the shortest length of time needed to treat the condition.
- Offer a naloxone prescription, especially if someone has risk factors for overdose. These include a history of substance use disorder, use of higher opioid dosages, previous overdoses, use of other sedating medications, or heart or breathing problems.
- Reevaluate, preferably face-to-face, the need for refills.
- Check urine drug screens (UDS) to make sure only the prescribed opioid is present.
- When prescribing long-term opioids, require face-to-face interaction at regular intervals, typically every three months, to evaluate whether symptoms have improved with opioid treatment, the goals of treatment and whether it is appropriate to slowly stop taking opioids, called tapering. Other discussion points include whether risk factors have changed and the risks and benefits of continuing to take opioids.

THE FOUNDATIONS FOR OPIOID PARTNERSHIP

Respect. If there's one word that describes the foundation for opioid safety, it's this one. Respect for the drugs, respect for the health care team and respect for the person taking the opioid.

Conversations surrounding opioids can be challenging for everyone involved, especially when expectations do not align.

Health care providers must balance managing their patients' pain and limiting negative effects, all while adhering to prescribing regulations.

People taking opioids must balance managing pain with the prescribing limitations needed for safe opioid use.

The opioid epidemic has shown that medicine should be a partnership, a commitment between health care providers and their patients. Both must commit to listen to each other, speak with honesty and agree to follow evidence-based science.

CREATING A HEALTHY PARTNERSHIP

The following chart shows some behaviors that promote a healthy partnership between people taking opioids and their health care providers.

People taking prescription opioids	Providers
Tell the truth	Listen carefully
Respect office policies	Ask questions without judgment
Use courteous language	Don't use stigmatizing language
Show respect to all office staff	Explain decisions in detail
Be receptive to challenging conversations	Answer with kindness and honesty
Be willing to try new solutions	Express empathy
Be patient	Be responsive to requests

An honest and respectful relationship allows people and providers to work together to achieve their goals.

OPIOID STORAGE AND DISPOSAL: BE SAFE!

Most people wouldn't dare keep drain cleaner within easy reach of their kids, so they take steps to make sure drain cleaner is safely stored. The same safety measures should apply to opioids.

For some people, the idea of keeping opioids close by and easy to access seems logical. After all, who wants to dig around when in pain?

But the epidemic has shown that in the wrong hands, these drugs can be deadly. Children are especially at risk. Studies show that more than 70% of people who use opioids for nonmedical reasons were able to get them from friends and family who didn't safely store or dispose of them.

Safe storage

Follow these guidelines for safe storage of opioids:
- Always keep the drugs in their original packaging or containers. Don't remove or change the label. Pill bottles and patch boxes contain vital information for managing these medications safely. Prescriptions always have patient-

identifying information so that health care providers can ensure medications are being taken by the right person. Prescription labels also have specific instructions on how the medication is intended to be used. Labels always note the dispensed amount of medication in the container.

- Think carefully about where you place bottles of opioids. Don't leave them on a counter or in a purse or a bag where someone else could easily get them.
- Keep opioids in a locked box or in a room inaccessible to teens, children, vulnerable adults and pets.
- Once you're done taking an opioid, get rid of the unused medication. Medications that have expired may not be effective or safe to take. And the longer the medications are around in the home, the more likely they'll be misused, either intentionally or by accident.

Safe disposal

Here's how to safely dispose of drugs containing opioids:

- Call your local city offices, police department or hospital to ask about 24/7 boxes (or drug take back locations) where you can drop off unused drugs.
- If you can't get to a drug take back location promptly, the FDA recommends that you flush drugs that contain opioids down the toilet. It's safer to do this than to keep them in your home.
- If you're not able to use these methods to dispose of opioid medication, remove the unused medication from the bottle and mix it with something that no person or animal wants to eat, such as

cat litter or coffee grounds. Place the mixture in a sealed plastic bag and throw the bag in the trash.

- You can also buy special bags that you can use to throw out medications called deactivation disposal bags (for example, Deterra). You can purchase them at many pharmacies.

A CAREFUL BALANCE

Opioids are a powerful pain management tool when used as part of an overall pain management plan — but using them requires a careful balance.

People taking opioids can feel empowered when they understand when and how to use opioids safely. Severe complications can be avoided by establishing a close partnership with providers and commitment to open, honest communication. With a healthy respect for opioids in place, the drugs can be the valuable tool they were meant to be and not the danger they sometimes become.

———— W H A T   I F ————

providers and patients try to understand each other's perspectives?

6

Opioid overdose: You can save a life

Even when opioids are taken properly, someone can still overdose. That's why it's important to be prepared.

Overdose is the most feared complication of taking opioids, and the rates of both fatal and nonfatal overdoses in America are rising. In fact, from 2005 to 2014, the number of emergency room visits due to opioid overdoses increased almost 100%. Although certain risk factors increase the chances of an opioid overdose, everyone is at risk. Even when taking opioids properly, someone can still overdose.

People taking opioids and those who spend time with them must be prepared. In this chapter, you'll learn about naloxone and how it can be used to save a life.

HOW DOES AN OVERDOSE HAPPEN?

An opioid overdose happens when opioids bind to receptors in the part of the brain that regulates breathing. The more opioid available to the brain, the higher the risk of overdosing.

An opioid overdose makes someone unable to breathe or maintain blood pressure and heart rate. Any of these can lead to death.

Overdoses can happen in people who take opioids for acute pain or chronic pain. They can happen when someone takes medically prescribed opioids or street drugs. People who take any type of opioid for any reason are at risk for overdosing, even accidentally.

A person overdosing on opioids may:
- Have very slow or irregular breathing. The person may appear to be sleeping but is struggling to breathe normally.
- Have a slow heartbeat. You may not be able to find a pulse at all.
- Have blue or gray edges around the mouth.
- Have blue fingernails.
- Have skin that is pale or gray and cool to the touch.
- Have very small pupils.
- Be sleepy or unresponsive.
- Be very confused.

Not everyone will have all these signs. Some people may have only one or two.

People at risk

The following actions increase the risk of overdosing:

- Taking higher doses of opioids.
- Taking opioids by injection.
- Taking medications that cause sleepiness at the same time as taking opioids. This includes a type of medication called benzodiazepines. Examples of benzodiazepines include diazepam (Valium), lorazepam (Ativan), clonazepam (Klonopin) and alprazolam (Xanax).
- Having a health condition that causes breathing problems. Examples of these include COPD, obstructive sleep apnea, interstitial lung disease and lung cancer.
- Having organ dysfunction such as liver or kidney disease that prevents the drug from being cleared from the body.
- Receiving treatment for opioid use disorder that includes medications.
- Having a history of substance or opioid use disorder.
- Having a mental health condition.
- Having overdosed from opioids in the past.

SHARE THIS INFORMATION!

If you overdose, it's unlikely that you'll be able to give yourself naloxone. For this reason, it's important that you share the information in this chapter and in Appendix F right away with:
- Caregivers.
- People who live with you.
- People who spend a lot of time with you.
- People who might be there during an emergency.

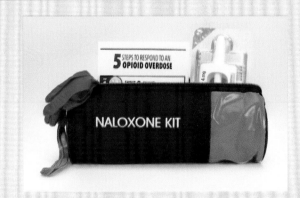

Understanding how to use naloxone before an overdose occurs may save a life — perhaps yours.

WHAT'S NALOXONE?

Naloxone is a prescription medication that quickly — but only temporarily — reverses an opioid overdose. Naloxone doesn't reverse an overdose from other medications.

Remember that naloxone is only a temporary solution to an overdose. It typically works for only 30 to 90 minutes. No matter which method you use to administer it, be prepared to give repeated doses as needed while you wait for emergency responders to arrive.

If you suspect someone is overdosing from an opioid, don't hesitate to give naloxone. **Give naloxone even if:**
- You don't know for certain the person is overdosing from an opioid. Giving naloxone to someone that hasn't overdosed from opioids won't hurt them.
- You think the overdose could be caused by an opioid mixed with other substances.
- You don't know whether the person is allergic to naloxone.

Don't worry about getting into legal trouble if you give someone naloxone. You're legally protected from this.

Follow these steps immediately if you suspect someone is overdosing from an opioid:
1. Call 911 or emergency medical help.
2. Check your surroundings to ensure you're safe. Look for traffic, needles, loose powder or other dangers.
3. Follow the directions given to you by the 911 or emergency medical help

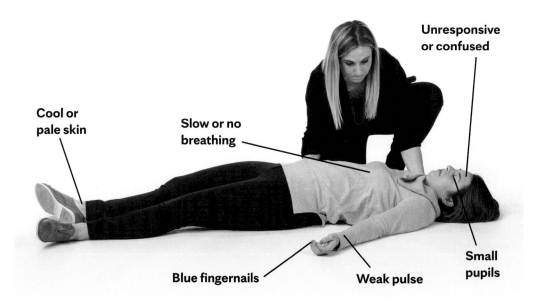

Signs of an opioid overdose

operator. This may include giving the person CPR if you're comfortable doing so.

4. Give naloxone.

You may hear naloxone called Narcan, which is a brand name of a naloxone product. You may also hear other brand names such as Kloxxado, Evzio or Zimhi. The naloxone brand and device you're given may be different from what's shown in the photos in Appendix F.

There are several ways to give naloxone, including using a nasal device to spray it in the nose or injecting it into a muscle. Follow the directions provided from your pharmacist and the manufacturer for your device.

Side effects of naloxone

Side effects of naloxone nasal spray include muscle pain and spasms; headache; dry, runny or stuffy nose; and constipation.

Side effects of injected naloxone include upset stomach, vomiting, dizziness, pain at the injection site and hot flashes.

Safe storage and disposal of naloxone

Follow the directions in Chapter 5 about how to safely store and dispose of any opioid, including naloxone.

In addition, follow these steps:
- Store naloxone at room temperature. Keep it out of direct light.
- If you gave someone naloxone using needles, place the needles in a hard-plastic container, such as an empty laundry detergent bottle. Ask your local waste collection company what to do with the bottle. Or once emergency responders arrive, ask them about how to safely dispose of the needles.
- Safely dispose of expired naloxone and ask for a new prescription.

One time I overdosed. The last thing I remember is giving myself heroin. Then I woke up with cops and paramedics around me and an ambulance outside my house. They gave me every dose of Narcan they had. I think it was six doses! One of the cops said, "You were dead, buddy." If they wouldn't have had Narcan, I wouldn't be here.

BRAD

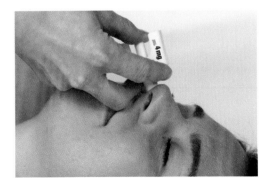

One of the most common ways to give naloxone is to spray it into the nose

KEEP YOURSELF SAFE

Before you give naloxone, look around at your surroundings. Make sure you're in a safe environment. If you suspect the overdose was due to a street drug, take extra care to protect yourself from touching any surfaces that may have been contaminated with the drug. Some street opioids can be very dangerous even when only touched. Consider using gloves if a pair is available.

When a person has been given naloxone and then wakes up, the person immediately goes into withdrawal and is likely to be very uncomfortable when waking up.

The person may:
- Act combatively and aggressively.
- Vomit, urinate, sweat, have diarrhea or be short of breath.
- Be confused, distressed or angry.

After you give someone naloxone, to keep yourself safe, move out of reach of the person right away.

A medical emergency

Remember that an opioid overdose is a medical emergency. Immediately call 911 or emergency medical help if you haven't already. Someone who has overdosed still needs immediate medical attention and must be seen by a health care provider right away. The person may have breathing problems that return within minutes of being given naloxone. The person's health care provider can determine next steps to prevent future overdose.

I call my son a miracle. He died two times. He was brought back. The right people were there at the right time to save him.

DIANA

IF YOU TAKE OPIOIDS

Think of using opioids like driving a car. Like a car, opioids can be of great value. But they can also cause a lot of damage if not used safely. Having naloxone on hand is that final click of the seat belt in case something goes wrong. Everyone prescribed an opioid should ask their provider if naloxone is right for them.

Follow these steps:
- Keep naloxone with you at all times.
- Make sure people you spend time with know how to give naloxone if needed.
- Consider wearing a medical alert bracelet that says you take an opioid.

Refer to Appendix F for how to administer naloxone using various methods. If you or those close to you have questions about when and how to use naloxone, contact your provider or a pharmacist.

——————— **WHAT IF** ———————

*your superpower can fit in
your back pocket?*

7

Hard-wired to feel: Understanding pain

For more than 200 years, prescription opioids have been a reliable tool for treating pain. To understand why the drugs work, it's key that you understand how the body creates pain and pain's overall purpose.

Unpleasant but protective, the point of pain is simple: It warns the body about active tissue injury. It's hard to imagine, but most times, pain comes to our rescue. It helps us set limits, prevents us from repeating mistakes and pushes us to seek help. When it works as it should, pain is a critical tool for our survival.

But what happens when pain becomes the disease? Pain can stop protecting and start manipulating. It can control your mood, job, relationships and productivity. It can inhibit the ability to participate in life itself. It can even change the way the body responds to opioids, turning pain-relief tools into agents of misery.

In this chapter, you'll learn how pain is created by the body and how, over time, pain can transition into its own disease.

THE VALUE OF PAIN

Your brain constantly receives information from your senses pertaining to temperature, touch, noise, sight, motion and taste. Your brain evaluates this incoming sensory information and, in response, sends signals to warn you of possible danger.

Imagine accidentally touching a hot stove. Your brain signals pain so that you pull your hand away from the stove. Your brain remembers that pain so that you're careful to avoid touching a hot stove in the future.

All pain you feel is part of this protection system. Pain motivates you to address a situation that may harm you and avoid repeating that situation, such as going near a hot stove the next time you are in the kitchen.

THE PROBLEM OF CHRONIC PAIN

Over time, however, pain can go from being protective to being a problem. Pain is called chronic when it lasts

HOW YOU FEEL PAIN

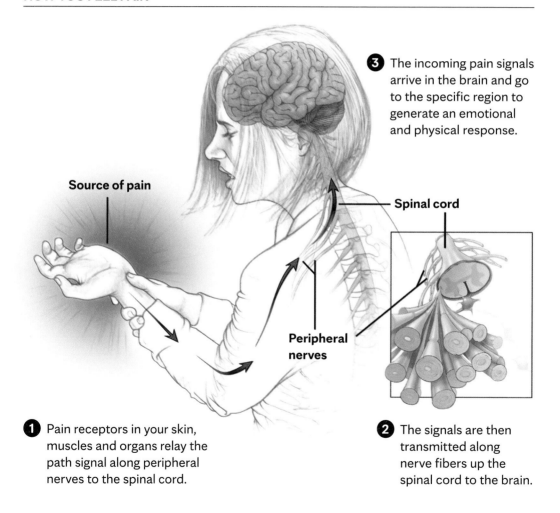

3 The incoming pain signals arrive in the brain and go to the specific region to generate an emotional and physical response.

Source of pain

Spinal cord

Peripheral nerves

1 Pain receptors in your skin, muscles and organs relay the path signal along peripheral nerves to the spinal cord.

2 The signals are then transmitted along nerve fibers up the spinal cord to the brain.

longer than a few months. Comparing acute pain to chronic pain is like comparing a lottery ticket to a traffic ticket: They may sound alike, but they're a world apart to the person holding one.

Unlike acute pain, which serves a protective purpose, chronic pain serves no purpose. In fact, chronic pain is a disease in itself. Pain that continues for months or years serves little function, and can prevent healing from taking place.

RISK FACTORS FOR DEVELOPING CHRONIC PAIN

Most people are about as enthusiastic about being in pain as they are about doing their taxes. A common goal is to keep chronic pain from developing in the first place.

Studies have shown that one of the most important risk factors for chronic pain is the degree of the initial pain itself. The more severe acute pain is, the greater the risk that the pain will become chronic.

This means there's enormous value in addressing pain at the time an injury occurs. For many people, if pain can be controlled in the acute phase, it can be prevented from transitioning to the chronic phase.

Many other factors affect the risk of developing chronic pain after an injury. Risk of chronic pain is greater if:
- You're older.
- You're a woman.
- You have a chronic inflammatory condition, such as rheumatoid arthritis or an inflammatory bowel disorder.
- You have a nerve-related condition. For example, people with diabetes often develop nerve damage (neuropathy), resulting in chronic pain in 60% of people with diabetes.

Unfortunately, there's no crystal ball to predict who will develop chronic pain and who won't. Two people who have the same injury may end up with very different outcomes.

If you experience an injury, the best way to avoid chronic pain is to take immediate action and focus on taking care of yourself. Also, have an honest discussion with your health care provider regarding pain treatment.

Sometimes chronic pain stems from an ongoing medically active disease like arthritis. With arthritis, persistent joint inflammation triggers repetitive nerve impulses and signals injury.

But chronic pain can also occur despite no obvious injury or disease. Also referred to as functional pain syndromes, examples include fibromyalgia, chronic daily headaches and irritable bowel syndrome. For each of these, standard laboratory tests, imaging and other medical tests fail to show disease.

Chronic pain syndromes are just as real as other medical conditions. They're debilitating. They can affect relationships. They can even affect quality of life.

According to the Institute of Medicine, chronic pain affects more Americans than cancer, heart disease and diabetes combined. In fact, it's estimated that up to 20% of all people suffer from some form of chronic pain.

LET'S TALK

Pain results from several lines of communication within the body. How does all this happen? The answer is the central nervous system.

The nervous system allows the different parts of your body to communicate. The human body contains special nerve cells called neurons. Neurons pick up information provided by your senses. This information is relayed to the central nervous system to be processed. The nervous system is always changing and adapting to the information coming in — for better or for worse.

Too much of a good thing

It's normal for brain structures and sensory pathways in the central nervous system to change in response to sensory input. This is called being neuroplastic. For most activities, neuroplasticity is a good thing. This ability to change can be helpful.

Think about taxi drivers in large cities, for instance. They have to learn to navigate various roads and intersections, remembering landmarks and finding alternate routes to avoid backups at peak traffic times. Over time, as more areas within the drivers' brains become involved in processing information about what they see, the drivers' brains become "hardwired" with alternative pathways to help them drive quickly and efficiently despite traffic and road construction.

Unfortunately, this ability to develop more pathways in the central nervous system can also create problems. As the brain begins to process incoming information from the senses faster, it creates more pathways to move sensory signals more efficiently — in some situations, too efficiently.

WHEN IT ALL GOES WRONG: CENTRAL SENSITIZATION

As the brain gets faster at processing sensory signals, it can become so sensitive to information that it can no longer accurately detect danger. The result is a central nervous system that interprets pain and other uncomfortable sensations as more intense than they really should be.

The central nervous system has become sensitized. Sensitization is like the volume control on a radio becoming stuck at high volume. Sensitization "turns up the volume" of pain messages, making them stronger and, at times, distorted. Sensitization can result in constant nausea, vomiting, fatigue, motion sickness (even at rest), dizziness and pain.

When someone has central sensitization, the brain overreacts to sensory signals — even ones that aren't painful — as if they're dangerous, uncomfortable and even painful. The central nervous system starts to use more areas to process information from the senses. This is called nerve recruitment, and it means brain neurons may recruit other nerves nearby to help process sensory information such as touch, movement, temperature and sound.

As these sensory signals travel through the nervous system, they become amplified. The more the pathways are activated, the easier it is for them to overreact to any signals from the senses. In time, even one sensory signal may activate many regions of the brain, causing widespread and more intense pain as well as other symptoms.

The brain's ability to improve efficiency is important when it comes to learning new skills. When someone practices the piano every day, more areas of the brain make

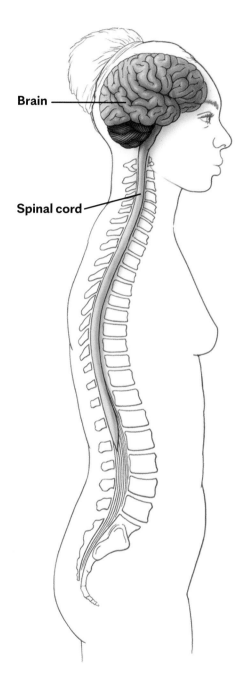

Brain

Spinal cord

The brain and spinal cord together comprise the central nervous system.

connections to help move fingers. In time, those finger movements become "hard-wired" in the brain of that person, who can then play almost without thinking. Unfortunately, the same process can occur with pain.

Health care providers can actually see nerve recruitment when they compare brain scans of people who don't have central sensitization with scans of those who do. In one study:

- When a heat probe was applied to the leg of people who didn't have central sensitization, the scans showed distinct activity in the area of the brain that recognizes sensory information.
- When a heat probe was applied to the leg of people who did have central sensitization, the scan showed larger areas of the brain involved in processing information, indicating more intense and widespread pain.

As the central nervous system becomes less accurate in processing sensory information, discomfort and pain become the automatic response. The body begins to perceive pain in an overly exaggerated manner through a condition called hyperalgesia. Things that usually hurt a little now hurt more. Even nerve impulses from a nonpainful stimulus, such as a light touch, can be perceived as pain. This extreme form of sensitization is a condition called allodynia.

If you have central sensitization, you may:

- Gag when you smell a strong odor.
- Feel like you're on a roller coaster when you ride in a car.
- Feel like your arm was wrenched out of its socket when all you did was move your shoulder.
- Feel like someone is shouting in your ear when someone only whispers to you.
- Feel like you've been awake for a week

Pain
No central sensitization

Pain
Central sensitization

The red and yellow areas in these illustrations show areas of brain activity. You can see that brain activity in response to pain increases in people who have central sensitization.

when only a couple of hours have passed since you woke up.

Why sensitization happens to some people and not to others is unknown. Factors that may play a role include:

- Injury or infection.
- Family history.
- Use of opioids for longer than 30 days.
- Poor sleep.
- Mental health problems, such as depression.
- Smoking.
- Trauma.
- Prolonged stress.
- Hormonal factors.
- Sex. Chronic pain is more common in women than men.

WHEN A SOLUTION BECOMES A PROBLEM

So, what's the connection between acute pain, chronic pain, central sensitization and opioids?

They are connected because many people seek out pain medications for relief from their pain. While opioids may help at first with acute pain, over time, the drugs provide less and less relief.

For people with chronic pain, opioids can become part of the problem instead of a solution. Research shows that opioids are generally not effective for most cases of long-term pain, and they can actually make chronic pain worse.

Taking opioids for chronic pain often leads to needing greater amounts of medication to manage the pain and, for some, opioid use disorder (OUD). To make the situation even more challenging, regular use of opioids can lead to tolerance. With tolerance, the pain may feel like it's getting worse over time when in fact the body isn't responding to opioids the same way that it used to.

Hyperalgesia

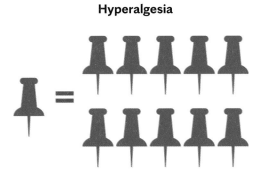

Allodynia

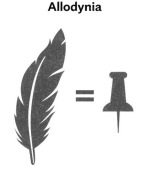

With hyperalgesia, one pushpin pricking you feels like 10 pushpins. With allodynia, even something as light as a feather can feel like a pushpin.

CHANGING YOUR LIFE IN THE FACE OF PAIN

Most people with chronic pain need to learn how to manage the pain without the use of opioids.

Remember how you read earlier that your brain is neuroplastic — it changes and adapts over time?

There are ways to retrain your brain so it can return to accurately processing information. With the right approach, you can help your brain process incoming information from your senses in a way that reduces your sensation of pain.

Harnessing the power of the autonomic nervous system

The autonomic nervous system is balanced by two branches: the sympathetic and parasympathetic.

You may be aware that the sympathetic branch is responsible for the stress response, often called the fight-or-flight response, which dictates the body's survival reactions to threat.

The sympathetic branch takes these actions in response to stress:
• Dilates pupils.
• Slows down saliva production.
• Increases heart rate.

LINDSEY: "IT'S JUST SIMPLE THINGS"

I worked in a kidney dialysis center and I spent long hours on my feet most of the day. That was hard on my back and knees. I would take opioids to numb the pain from this. I used opioids for about 10 years.

Then I read a book about how pain works. It helped me understand the pain network. I learned pain is a warning signal that something is wrong.

In today's society, it seems like everyone wants a quick fix to get the outcome they want. But after reading that book, I learned pain is kind of necessary; it might be telling you that something is wrong.

I learned that opioids weren't the only answer. They were just a crutch. They weren't solving my pain problem; they were just numbing it. They weren't helping me live a better life, a pain-free life.

I learned there are other therapies that could help relieve some of the pain. In treatment, I'm learning how to live without dependence on opioids. Been sober 11 months now! I'm getting a lot of plain exercise and doing different stretches. I'm doing yoga, which helps my back. It's just simple things I'm doing but they really help.

- Turns off digestive tract.
- Stimulates adrenaline production.
- Promotes urination.

When the sympathetic branch is in control for longer than necessary, it creates chronic wear and tear on the body's organs and systems, creating a sensitized nervous system.

The parasympathetic branch initiates the "rest-and-digest" relaxation response. It calms the body so it can perform daily activities. It turns down the volume on stress and allows the brain to process information more accurately.

The parasympathetic branch takes these actions in response to stress:
- Constricts pupils.
- Increases saliva production.
- Reduces heart rate.
- Activates digestive tract.
- Prevents urination.

If you have central sensitization, you need to strengthen the parasympathetic branch of your nervous system and use

SOOTHE YOUR NERVOUS SYSTEM

Here are some strategies to help you activate the parasympathetic branch of your nervous system. Some health care providers call it "soothing the central nervous system."

Helpful behaviors
- Slowed breathing.
- Meditation or deep prayer.
- Imagery, visualizing a calm, peaceful, safe, healing place.
- Gentle yoga or tai chi.
- Daily physical activity.
- Daily stretching exercises.
- Healthy sleep habits.
- Change in pain thoughts and behaviors.

Behaviors that aren't helpful
- Thinking about pain all the time.
- Too much focus on symptom relief and not enough on regaining function.
- Fear of physical activity to the point of not moving at all.
- Using pain behaviors to draw attention.
- Pain catastrophizing — irrationally negative thoughts about pain, such as "This pain in my neck will never get better."

My son Vincent had so much life in him. He could have been anything in life. But rather than live with terrible pain, he chose to end it his own way.

Everyone said he was the funniest and most outgoing person they knew. There is no one he wouldn't help. He was intelligent and the class president of his high school. He was a tutor at Harvard and working on his doctorate at Penn State. He was preparing for a life of leadership in international business. The world was at his fingertips. But it all came crashing down after a freak accident that caused a head injury.

Vincent didn't tell us about it at first. He went to his health care provider to get help, but the treatments she offered didn't seem to make a difference.

Things got worse. He lost his ability to focus on his research and on anything else for that matter. His life started to deteriorate. He couldn't work out anymore, couldn't ride his bike or drive long distances.

He wanted help but didn't know where to turn. He felt like the medical system he trusted was letting him down. He didn't know how to navigate it or what kinds of questions to ask.

His treatment plan wasn't working and his life was changing.

Vincent came home for a weekend visit and he finally shared his struggles with us, his family. I'm a nurse. I understand pain and I know how debilitating it is. I knew enough to know he needed help — and needed it quickly. What I didn't know was that he couldn't take the pain even one day more. Shortly after he arrived home, he mentioned he was going to take a quick trip downtown.

A few hours later, there was a knock at my door. A police officer was standing there. He told me that my son had been found and the outcome was not good. I fell to my knees and started screaming, "NO, NO, NO, not my boy, not my son!"

There are no words to describe the feelings in those moments, those days following and even now.

As the police described to me what happened in the minutes before he died, I kept thinking, "That was my son." And other times, I'd think, "That was not my son."

strategies that put the parasympathetic branch back in control. The goal is to retrain your brain to react more appropriately to sensory input, reducing pain and other symptoms caused by central sensitization.

TAKE CONTROL

Talk to your health care provider about pain after injuries. If you have chronic or debilitating pain, tell someone who cares about you — someone who can go with you to appointments and speak up on your behalf.

Ask your provider about referral to a pain management program, also known as pain rehabilitation programs. These programs use behavioral, physical and occupational therapies to help you learn to manage chronic pain without the use of opioids. You can turn the devastation of pain into a destination of healing — and most importantly, prevent opioids from taking over your life.

For some people, pain can be so debilitating that it contributes to thoughts of suicide. If you're thinking about suicide, tell a loved one right away and call 988, the National Suicide Prevention Lifeline.

─────── **WHAT IF** ───────

we choose to not allow pain to be in control?

─────────────────────

IF YOU'RE THINKING ABOUT SUICIDE

Call 988 or 800-273-8255 to connect with the National Suicide Prevention Lifeline.

Or

Text HOME to 741741 (Crisis Text Line) to connect with a crisis counselor.

Evaluating pain and managing it safely

8

Take a moment to ask yourself: What would life be like if pain didn't control your thoughts and behaviors? What would life feel like free from the opioids used to manage that pain?

If you're one of the millions of Americans who lives with chronic pain and uses opioids to manage it, these are questions you likely ask yourself all the time.

Researchers estimate that from 40% to 70% of people with chronic pain don't receive proper medical treatment, which includes both under- and overtreating the pain. The more health care providers understand chronic pain, the more they've learned that "less is more" when it comes to opioids: more function, more quality of life and more time free from pain.

In this chapter, we explore the keys to setting and achieving reasonable pain treatment goals as well as the treatment tools to keep pain manageable.

Be careful when you take an opioid. You might find you like it. You might be one of those people who really digs it. Get off them as soon as you can. If you can, find another way to deal with your pain.

BRAD

ESTABLISHING REASONABLE TREATMENT GOALS

Ask any person in pain what their primary goal is and a likely response is "no more pain."

Pain prevents. It keeps us from taking part in activities and enjoying relationships. It dampens the joy and excitement of life's most memorable moments. Pain causes moment-to-moment misery that prevents people from living well. But is it possible to eliminate pain entirely? And will doing so help you live more fully?

As it turns out, the science says the answer may be no. The opioid epidemic sheds light on a powerful truth related to these questions: The absence of pain doesn't necessarily mean the presence of a good life.

In the early and mid-2000s, well-meaning attempts by health care providers to eliminate pain required increasing the dose of opioids or other sedating drugs, often to unhealthy levels. These higher doses accomplished the opposite of the providers' intent.

Instead of freeing people, the drugs imprisoned them. People struggled with lethargy and fear of withdrawal symptoms. They lived dose-to-dose, afraid of their pain returning. The solution — opioids — had become the problem. But how bad was the pain problem?

In seeking a way to assess and communicate about pain, both health care providers and people in pain have become very focused on the numbers on a scale.

What exactly is a pain scale?

You've probably heard something like this: "On a scale of 0 to 10 — with 0 being no pain and 10 being that guy who got eaten in 'Jurassic Park' — how would you rate your pain?"

"It's an 8," you may have responded.

Pain scales are a communication tool, a way to tell a health care provider about pain. They offer a way to assign a value to a relatively subjective experience. This value gives providers a rough idea of how one person's pain fits into a range of extremes.

Unfortunately, these pain scales don't account for a person's tolerance for pain or the emotional drivers that can increase it. For some people, even though they rank their pain at an 8, they can run a marathon, while others cannot get out of bed with a score of 3.

Other pain assessment tools are based on descriptors, such as pain location, how severe the pain is, whether it spreads from one place to another and when it happens. Pain scales don't account for various aspects of pain, and the descriptions are hard to compare between people. Pain scales need to be paired with more objective information. They need context.

Imagine trying to use numbers to describe the colors of a painting, the aroma of chicken soup or how it feels to watch a sunset. Numbers can't appropriately represent the subjective qualities needed to describe each of these.

These examples demonstrate the inherent problem of only using number scales to assess pain and determine the success of treatments. Number scales fail to address how pain impacts people's ability to engage in daily activities.

As a result, providers are transitioning away from using only pain scores and descriptors to monitor pain and treatment success. Pain scores and descriptors play an important role in pain assessment, but they're no longer the only tools used.

The new focus of pain management has become good function and quality of life.

Providers are now striving to assess the person, not the number. They are asking people what's important to them. Is it being able to go to work? Sitting at a dinner table with family? Having water balloon fights with the grandkids?

Answering these questions has helped people communicate about their pain more effectively than using just a number.

This profound change in thinking has put the person with pain at the center of the discussion, not just the pain.

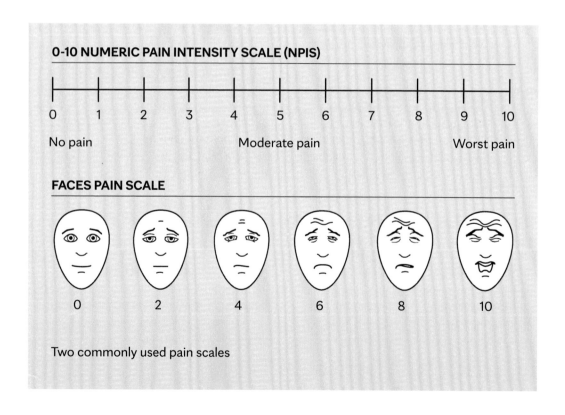

0-10 NUMERIC PAIN INTENSITY SCALE (NPIS)

0   1   2   3   4   5   6   7   8   9   10

No pain   Moderate pain   Worst pain

FACES PAIN SCALE

0   2   4   6   8   10

Two commonly used pain scales

For some people, elimination of pain may still be realistic. Medications, interventional procedures and activities such as physical therapy have helped many improve their quality of life.

To help find the right approach for you, your health care provider may ask you:
- What makes your pain worse? What makes it better?
- How would you describe the pain? Is it sharp, stabbing, dull, throbbing, burning, aching or something else?
- Where do you feel the pain? Does it spread from one place to another?
- How bad is the pain? What does the pain prevent you from doing?
- When does the pain come on? What triggers it? How long does it last?
- What treatments have been tried for the pain? Did they work?

SETTING THE RECORD STRAIGHT

If every person experienced pain the same way, there would be a single solution to the problem. But the reality is that people feel pain differently, and perception of pain can change from day to day. Pain may get better with certain activities and get worse with others. It increases and decreases with the time of day, with certain emotions and even with what's for dinner.

Given that so many variables can affect the experience of pain, it's important to monitor which factors have the greatest impact. Then health care providers can create treatment plans that offer the greatest chance of success.

Keep a pain journal

Let's face it: Not all of us were great in English class. Not all of us even went to English class. But the value of putting pen to paper — or fingertips to keyboard — cannot be overstated when it comes to understanding pain and helping create an effective treatment plan. A clear record of details about a person's pain can be an invaluable tool.

Journaling is often not only a form of therapy in itself but also a tremendous resource to capture potential pain triggers, patterns and responses to treatment.

Important items to track include:
- Severity.
- Timing of onset.
- Frequency of flare-ups.
- What makes pain worse or better.
- Response to treatments.

Of course, "There's an app for that." Digital trackers, which are widely available, can help keep you on track with prompts and reminders. Some apps can even help detect pain patterns and allow you to share information with others, such as your health care provider.

PAIN MANAGEMENT OPTIONS

Where would the world be without pain medications? If you ask the more than 70% of people annually who choose to use an epidural during childbirth, a likely answer is, "Still pregnant!"

To relieve suffering is a cornerstone of medical care. A significant amount of research has been spent developing new treatment options for pain. These include interventions and procedures, medications and mind-body therapies.

Although many conditions seem to respond well to certain treatments, no single treatment works for every person. Health care providers may need to work through a variety of treatments to identify what brings pain relief to someone. In addition, as disorders change or progress over time, some therapies may stop working and require transitions to other types of treatments.

Regardless of what treatment plan someone has been given, the key to success is setting realistic goals. Knowing that easing pain doesn't mean taking it away completely can set the stage for successful goal setting.

The ultimate goal of treatment is to manage symptoms so that people can go about their activities of daily living while enjoying a good quality of life.

Many treatments can take weeks to deliver the full effect. Your health care provider can let you know when to expect some pain relief and what alternatives should be used in the meantime.

Remember, acute pain that persists beyond the usual time of healing may turn into chronic pain. Chronic pain requires different treatments from those used for acute pain.

If someone came in my office right now who had chronic pain and was taking high levels of opioids, I'd say, "I understand you got put on this level of morphine for good reason. But we have evidence that suggests that you might actually be feeling more pain now than you would be if we weren't using opioids at all."

Then I draw a little diagram and show them how their pain goes up and down, but it would be up and down at a lower level without the opioids. I tell them we are going to find other ways to manage their pain.

DR. MATT DAY,
HEALTH CARE PROVIDER AND ADDICTION SPECIALIST

In Chapter 7, you read how chronic pain may be associated with central sensitization, where pain is more intense than would be expected. In these circumstances, providers may use medications that calm the central nervous system combined with brain retraining therapies that do not involve medication.

The information that follows describes treatment options that don't involve opioids. Read about how these options may be used alone or in combination to treat pain and how opioids may be part of the equation when used by the right person, for the right reason, in the right form, at the right dose and for the right length of treatment.

Nonopioids with powerful potency

Evidence from research on the powerful pain-controlling properties of nonopioid medications continues to grow. For most people, these medications are safer to use than opioids. Health care providers may recommend their use in combination or with other nondrug therapies for both acute and chronic pain. Below are some common opioid alternatives with powerful pain-relieving effects.

Acetaminophen

Though not as strong as most opioids, acetaminophen (Tylenol) has shown good results in pain management. It can be used for both acute and chronic pain, particularly when chronic pain has an inflammatory cause.

Acetaminophen has also been shown to reduce the need for opioids. It is particularly useful as first-line pain relief after an injury or surgery, often in combination with nonsteroidal anti-inflammatory drugs (NSAIDs). People taking it must limit their total daily dosage to no more than 4,000 mg/day to avoid liver problems. If you are taking acetaminophen, do not drink alcohol.

Nonsteroidal anti-inflammatory drugs

NSAIDs are a class of medications that reduce fever, inflammation and pain.

They regulate inflammatory proteins in the blood as well as some aspects of blood clotting. Examples of medications in this class include aspirin, naproxen (Aleve), ibuprofen (Advil, Motrin) and the prescription NSAIDs diclofenac and ketorolac.

Similar to acetaminophen, these drugs work well to treat acute pain and can help reduce the need to take opioids. For most people without a prior history of medical issues, the drugs can be used safely for short periods of time. If you are going to take NSAIDs, talk with your provider first. Medical conditions such as kidney disease or stomach ulcers can develop or worsen when taking these drugs.

COX-2 inhibitors

COX-2 inhibitors are a class of medications that selectively inhibit the COX-2 enzyme, which reduces overall inflammation. The benefit of these prescription drugs is that they are taken once or twice daily and provide long-lasting pain relief. They're excellent treatment strategies for chronic pain when the pain is caused by inflammation, such as arthritis. The only available COX-2 inhibitor currently available in the U.S. is celecoxib.

Gabapentinoids

Unlike the other drugs listed here, gabapentinoids work primarily by reducing inappropriate nerve conduction. They're typically used only for certain painful conditions designated as neuropathic pain.

This class of medications includes the drugs gabapentin and pregabalin. These drugs might be used to treat conditions such as diabetic neuropathy or chemotherapy-induced nerve pain. Studies have shown that some people can develop breathing problems when these medications are taken with opioids or taken by people over a certain age or with liver and kidney problems.

Antidepressants

Don't be turned off by the name of this class of drugs. Evidence shows antidepressants can be used for more than just depression. These medications affect the processing and signaling of neurotransmitters that regulate both mood and pain sensations. They've been particularly helpful for several chronic pain conditions, such as fibromyalgia and migraine headaches.

Health care providers sometimes prescribe them for people who are beginning to taper off opioids.

Examples of antidepressants include tricyclic antidepressants, selective serotonin reuptake inhibitors and serotonin-norepinephrine reuptake inhibitors.

Steroids

Since inflammation is a driver of pain, strong anti-inflammatory medications can suppress the body's immune response to injury. Steroids have been shown to reduce acute pain after surgery and other injuries. They include drugs such as dexamethasone, prednisone and prednisolone.

DARREN: "THAT WAS NOT A GOOD CHOICE"

My opioid addiction started when I was given pain meds after getting four wisdom teeth pulled. They prescribed me Vicodin. I loved the feeling it gave me. So that was not a good choice for relieving my pain. I should have stayed with ibuprofen.

Then I got a bad cold and I got prescribed a cough syrup with codeine. So I decided to see how I would feel with the cough syrup mixed with Vicodin. Then I really got addicted to opioids.

Today, I am sober from opioids going on three and a half years. I am sober because I got treatment from a great program. I've learned that pain may come but it is only temporary.

I can't go to opioids. I've learned other pain meds like ibuprofen may not work as well but are safer ways to ease physical pain and avoid addiction. Opioids are very addictive.

Steroids carry several side effects and can cause long-term health problems, such as weight gain, diabetes and other problems. For this reason, steroids are typically only prescribed for very short periods of time. Sometimes, they're given one time during a procedure.

Topical medications

Topical medications are applied to the skin. If the source of pain is close to the outside of the body — such as with muscle and joint pain or superficial skin pain — topical medications can be helpful.

One example is a topical anesthetic called lidocaine. Lidocaine patches are applied close to the source of pain. Lidocaine is also available in a cream and ointment form. Another topical drug is capsaicin, which is derived from chili peppers, available to buy without a prescription. It's made into an ointment or patch.

Topical nonsteroidal anti-inflammatory agents, such as diclofenac (Voltaren), have also proven effective in treating inflammatory conditions, such as osteoarthritis.

Interventional medical procedures

In certain situations, interventional medical procedures can be a valuable tool in the treatment of pain. Interventional procedures work either by targeting the painful body part directly or by targeting the nerve supply to the painful structure or body part.

The table on page 96 lists many common interventional procedures used to treat pain. Most often, interventional procedures are combined with other treatments, such as physical therapy, exercise or oral medications. Combining these with other treatments increases the likelihood of good symptom control.

GET MOVING

When in pain, it's natural to want to slow down. But studies show limiting movement can actually make pain worse. A common phrase in medicine is, "Weakness creates more weakness." This means that doing nothing with the body only makes the body feel worse and weaker.

Of course, if pain is originating from an injury that needs time to heal, it's important to protect that part of the body. This list includes suggestions about how to stay active when dealing with painful conditions.

- **Aerobic exercise** includes activities that increase heart rate and improve cardiovascular health. Examples include walking, cycling and swimming. Aerobic activity benefits the heart, lungs and circulatory system. It also improves cognitive function and stamina for daily activities. Aerobic activity has been shown to decrease stress, improve the ability to digest food and drink, ease depression and anxiety and manage chronic pain.
- **Strength training** involves contracting muscles against resistance using free weights, elastic bands, water resistance or personal body weight. Strength

INTERVENTIONAL PROCEDURES

Procedure	Description	Examples of treatment
Joint injection	Injections are given to treat joint pain and inflammation.	Knee joint, hip joint, shoulder joint, spinal facet joint pain and bursitis.
Radiofrequency ablation	A heated probe or special needle is used to deaden, or ablate, nerve endings to painful body areas or structures.	Spine pain from facet joints, knee pain, hip pain or shoulder pain. Can also be used to treat or ablate painful tumors.
Cryoablation	A probe or special needle is used to freeze or deaden nerve endings to painful body areas or structures.	Painful tumors.
Prolotherapy	Medication is injected around damaged ligaments and tendons to induce tissue healing.	Tennis elbow, sacroiliac ligament injury, knee and ankle ligament sprains.
Platelet-rich plasma injection (PRP)	This treatment is experimental. Injections are given of the platelet concentrate from a person's own blood into a painful joint or tendon to promote healing.	Knee degenerative arthritis, spinal joint arthritis, tendon injuries, such as Achilles tendonitis and plantar fasciitis.
Stem cell injection	This treatment is experimental. It involves taking a person's own stem cells and injecting them into damaged joint or tendon tissue to promote healing.	Knee degenerative arthritis; spinal joint arthritis; tendon injuries, such as Achilles tendonitis and plantar fasciitis; degenerative disk pain.
Spinal cord and peripheral nerve stimulation (SCS, PNS, TENS)	Medical device consisting of a wire lead and a generator (battery). Some devices are surgically implanted near a nerve or the spinal cord. Others are placed on the skin. They electrically block or modulate pain signals.	Severe spinal pain or limb pain, or both, that has not responded to medications, physical therapy or surgery.
Drug pump or intrathecal drug delivery device	Medical device with a flexible tube connected to a small drug pump. The device is surgically implanted to deliver potent pain medications directly to the spinal canal.	Severe cancer-related pain or spinal pain that has not responded to less invasive therapy.

training can reduce fatigue, support joints and increase strength and stamina.

- **Flexibility training** includes exercises meant to improve joint range of motion and reduce stiffness.
- **Physical therapy** focuses on exercises and physical activities, such as massage, applying heat and ice, and limb manipulation. Physical therapy can promote movement and restore function.
- **Occupational therapy** focuses on understanding a person's abilities and limitations to help the person adapt to the environment.

THE POWER OF POSITIVITY

For many people, pain is overwhelming and managing it becomes the focus of living. Having a positive attitude, turning the focus away from pain and calming negative emotions can have powerful effects.

A large study found that inactive substances, commonly referred to as placebo pills, relieved pain just as well as medications themselves in up to half of the study participants. The study concluded that the human brain responds well to positive thinking. By just being told that they would experience improvement, participants did experience an improvement.

What your brain expects

One study investigated how people perceive pain on the basis of what they thought pain would actually feel like.

Study participants had a small electrode placed on them that was set to a temperature of 120 degrees Fahrenheit.

One set of participants were shown an image that suggested the pain they were about to experience would be severe. The second set of participants were shown an image that suggested the pain would be tolerable.

The electrode was heated up briefly, giving the same sensation to both groups. Participants ranked the severity of the pain they experienced. Magnetic resonance imaging (MRI) brain scans were done as well.

Those who were shown the image of severe pain scored the pain as worse compared with those who were shown the image of tolerable pain. In other words, after the brain received a cue that the pain would be severe, it acted as though the pain were severe.

The researchers concluded that the brain responds on the basis of what it expects to feel, and multiple studies have shown that the power of placebos lies in the brain's expectation that an effect will happen.

Given these results, is it possible that positive thinking can support healing or lessen pain?

Brain imaging scans have confirmed that placebos can activate the same brain pathways that medications typically trigger. This isn't meant to suggest that placebos should be a treatment, but it does shine light on the potential power of having a positive outlook when it comes to pain management.

Integrative therapies

Recognizing the power of the mind when it comes to pain management, scientists have looked at various mind-body treatments, also known as integrative therapies, as potential options for pain management. Integrative therapies target the mind-body connection of symptoms and often include practices that were not traditionally part of Western medicine.

Many integrative therapies focus on creating a state of calm within the body. Relaxation helps reduce the sympathetic fight-or-flight response in the body and promotes the parasympathetic rest-and-digest state. Many integrative therapies help people recognize which of these two states their bodies are in.

Integrative therapies have been used successfully to help people reduce the amount of medication they take. These therapies have been so successful that many are now endorsed by government health agencies, such as the Centers for Disease Control and Prevention, and major medical organizations. Insurance companies cover many of these options.

Hospital regulatory organizations now require accredited hospitals and clinics to offer them.

COMBINING OPIOIDS WITH OTHER TREATMENTS

The opioid epidemic has shown that there's virtually no role for a pain treatment plan that only includes opioids. There are always opportunities to combine opioids with other treatments. These may include other nonopioid medications, interventional or topical treatments, physical activity and integrative therapies. There are several reasons why using multiple approaches at once offers the best pain management.

First, people taking only opioids may have pain relief but usually for only four to six hours. This leaves them at risk of gaps in pain control when the medication's effects begin to wear off but it's not yet time for the next dose.

Second, the cause of someone's pain may be related to trauma, inflammation or even rewiring of the brain. Because opioids target only one main pathway of pain development, it's important to include other pain management tools for effective treatment. These additional tools target other pathways, such as inflammation, that drive the pain response. The key is to address the total pain experience.

Using tools in the toolbox

Most providers recommend trying multiple treatments at the same time. Often, combining multiple medications or medications and nonmedication treatments offers

EXAMPLES OF INTEGRATIVE THERAPIES

A number of integrative therapies can be used to help manage chronic pain and reduce the need for medications:

- **Cognitive behavioral therapy (CBT).** CBT is a form of psychotherapy used to treat chronic pain based on the principle that thoughts, feelings and behaviors work together to influence overall well-being. The goal of CBT is for people to learn how to manage their unhealthy thoughts, feelings and behaviors that make central sensitization worse.

- **Biofeedback.** Biofeedback is a mind-body technique that stems from the theory that anything that can be measured can be changed. During a biofeedback session, sensors are connected to the skin and used to measure variations in vital signs, brain activity, breathing patterns or muscle tension. These are all body functions that can change during stress or pain. This information is fed back to the person, "closing the loop" of communication through a beeping sound or flashing light on a monitor to help the person change behaviors. The goal of biofeedback is to help a person recognize their body's responses to stress, anxiety, pain and chronic symptoms. Biofeedback can show which relaxation techniques are the most helpful to work on.

- **Spirituality.** Spirituality is the experience of transcendence or a connectedness to a greater purpose or power in life. Engaging in spiritual practices can calm anxiety, provide perspective and help bring a sense of purpose and resolve.

- **Yoga.** Yoga is a mind-body practice that combines breathing techniques and meditation with poses designed to stretch and strengthen muscles, improve physical fitness, enable relaxation, induce stress relief and lessen pain.

- **Massage therapy.** Massage therapy uses systematic rubbing and manipulation of body parts to reduce muscle tension and stress, treat pain, promote relaxation and create a feeling of general well-being.

- **Acupuncture.** Acupuncture is a traditional Chinese practice that involves inserting thin needles at certain places, called acupoints. This is done to alleviate pain and nerve tension. Acupuncture is believed to increase the body's natural ability to fight pain and to affect brain chemicals and hormones related to blood pressure, blood flow, temperature and the immune system.

- **Deep breathing.** Deep breathing creates relaxation in the body by reducing the sympathetic response and increasing the parasympathetic response. These are also called abdominal breathing exercises. The technique involves slowly and repetitively breathing air in and out using the diaphragm.

the best chance for relief. Providers sometimes call this list of treatment options a toolbox. And like hammers and nails or drills and bits, some tools work best when combined with others.

Providers can carefully consider which tools to use. Some pain disorders share similar signaling pathways and neurotransmitters, making their response to treatments somewhat predictable. Providers can use this background information, as well as clinical studies and personal experiences, to create the best pain management plan for each person.

People who take opioids for longer periods should always be treated with a combination approach involving other therapies. For many people, these will include:
- Medications, such as gabapentinoids or antidepressants.
- Interventional procedures, such as joint injections.
- Integrative therapies.
- Activities that keep the body moving.

TAKING PAIN MEDICATION ON A SCHEDULE

People who are offered opioids for acute pain relief should consider using acetaminophen or NSAIDs on a scheduled basis. People should avoid taking opioids unless needed for breakthrough pain.

Including more than one medication on a schedule makes it possible to take a medication every one to four hours for pain. Keeping a written schedule can help people stay on track.

Here is an example of a pain-management medication schedule for acute moderate to severe pain*:
- 8 a.m. — Acetaminophen (1,000 mg)
- 12 p.m. — Ibuprofen (200 mg)
- 1 p.m. — Oxycodone (2.5 mg) if needed for breakthrough pain
- 4 p.m. — Acetaminophen (1,000 mg)
- 8 p.m. — Ibuprofen (200 mg)
- 10 p.m. — Acetaminophen (1,000 mg)
- 11 p.m. — Oxycodone (2.5 mg) if needed for breakthrough pain

*This is just an example. Talk with your health care provider before you begin a schedule like this. Some people with certain health conditions should not take acetaminophen or ibuprofen.

Trial and error

Not all treatments work for all people. Not all treatments work right away. It's not unusual for someone to go through a series of treatments before finding a plan that works — one that leads to the greatest pain relief with the least side effects. This is especially true for people who have chronic pain.

Many health care providers recommend trying a treatment plan for two to three months. And they often ask people to record their pain experiences in a journal, answering questions such as:
• Did the method work?
• Were there side effects?
• When did the pain return?

The provider then uses that information to make decisions going forward. If pain management goals aren't achieved after two to three months, the provider and patient can create another plan.

FOCUS ON THE PERSON, NOT THE DISEASE

Changing how health care providers think about pain management has put the *person* in pain at the center of treatment goals.

Indeed, the most important goal of pain management is the health, safety and well-being of those dealing with pain. The road to get there may look different for each person, but all should reach the same destination — living a better life with less pain. With the list of treatment options growing every year, this life becomes more attainable every day.

——— **WHAT IF** ———

we commit to treating the person instead of just the pain?

DAVID: "I WAS SO RELIEVED"

I grew up on a Christmas tree farm in Iowa. I had a great childhood. My uncle and I did a lot of farming together and it was really good. I developed a strong work ethic, working hard and spending time outside. When I went to college, I changed majors a couple times but finally settled on horticulture, then I started my own landscaping business. I worked all the time, but everything was good.

Then I had a bad accident at work. I was in the hospital for weeks and in a wheelchair for months. I was having surgery about once every six months because they would fix something and then find something else.

I had so much pain from it all. From the beginning, they were giving me opioids. At first, the pills worked, but then I found that one pill didn't help, so I took two. I'd run out before I was due for a refill so I'd find ways to get more. I couldn't stop taking them because I'd feel so awful from the withdrawal symptoms. I was spending thousands of dollars to buy pills.

In the back of my mind, I knew that something was wrong. I knew I was addicted. Your body and your mind switch into this animal instinct to protect yourself. You'll find ways to try to get the pills. That's all you can think about. I knew things were bad, but I didn't know how to get out of it.

My family did an intervention. I wasn't mad about that. My wife, dad, brother and a friend were there. I wasn't upset they did this — I was so relieved.

My biggest fear wasn't about getting treatment: It was about letting everyone down. So I stopped taking the opioids cold turkey. It was the most miserable seven days of my life. I didn't understand at the time that I could have gotten help for the withdrawal symptoms.

Treatment helped me get over my worries of letting people down. It helped me with lots of things. I stayed in the program because I wanted to prove to my family that I could do it. My family and friends were very supportive. I don't know if I'd be here today without that support.

I understand what would happen if I relapsed. There are little temptations every day, but I don't let them take over. I know that I can only control me. I've had more surgeries since I got sober, but I find other ways to deal with pain. I'd rather deal with pain than go through all that again.

My advice to others is get treatment. If you find yourself getting off track, get help again. Go to the meetings you should go to. Do what your treatment program counselors tell you to do. I've been sober a long time and I plan to stay that way. I've come a long way.

DAVID'S WIFE: "I DIDN'T UNDERSTAND ADDICTION LIKE I DO NOW"

David and I got married about three years after his accident. I knew he was taking pain pills on and off, but I didn't know how much or what he was doing to get them.

Then I realized he had become addicted. I knew this because he couldn't wait until the next time he could take them. His behavior changed from the man I thought I knew. He wanted to just lie down all the time and he didn't want to spend time with our family.

He was so good at acting like he had things under control. I just had no idea. I kept thinking everything was going well. But we always seemed short of money and I didn't know where the money was going. One day I went to the bank and asked for a printout of our account. My son and I went through it together and we could see a bunch of ATM withdrawals, like $400 here and there on the same day. I knew then things were very bad.

We decided to do an intervention. We said, "David, we know what you are doing. We know you are taking pills." Amazingly, he said, "Yes, I am." He seemed relieved that it was out in the open! He said, "I don't want to live like this anymore."

I was bawling. I felt betrayed, lied to. I felt sick with this terrible feeling in my gut and I cried a lot. I didn't understand addiction like I do now.

Our family doctor said to go to the ER. This was a long while ago and back then, people at the ERs didn't know what to do with people like my husband. They just sent us home with a few suggestions and a pamphlet. That was a very bad day. We felt like we just had no hope.

But David's dad didn't give up. He did lots of research and found a treatment program for David. This treatment program was the best thing ever. My daughter and I went to therapy too.

David has been sober ever since. I have no doubt of that. We never gave up. Going through something like this makes you appreciate the small things in life. David has come a long way. We've all come a long way.

Opioid use disorder

 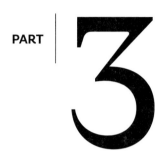

Understanding addiction and opioid use disorder

Addiction to opioids, also known as opioid use disorder (OUD), is one of the most challenging complications of opioid use. Affecting more than 2 million people in the U.S. alone, the condition is estimated to affect 3% to 19% of people using prescription opioids. More than two-thirds of all drug overdoses in the U.S. involve an opioid. Having OUD is a major risk factor for overdosing on opioids.

With statistics this sobering, prevention and treatment of OUD becomes one of the most important topics we as a nation must address.

Managing OUD requires that we understand its roots. What drives addiction? Is it a biological problem or a mental health disorder? Is anyone taking an opioid at risk for developing OUD, or is it just a concern for people with certain risk factors? What does OUD look like when it develops? Can friends and family see signs of it developing in early stages?

In this chapter, we break down the true causes of addiction and discuss the importance of early identification, treatment and opioid stewardship in preventing OUD.

WHAT IS DRUG ADDICTION?

Drug addiction is a chronic condition in which people use substances or engage in drug-related activities to the point that they have difficulty controlling their behavior. In some people, the disorder is obvious because addiction can impact many parts of someone's life.

It may manifest as a friend's son living on the streets and stealing from family to afford heroin. Health care providers may recognize it in someone visiting multiple emergency rooms each month, reporting various complaints in attempts to obtain opioid prescriptions.

In some situations, the disorder can be silent, an unrecognized and very personal experience. Perhaps someone is driven by unbearable emotional pain due to childhood trauma to seek relief by sneaking an oxycodone from a family member.

Or perhaps a person who was originally prescribed opioids for a legitimate chronic medical condition now wants to use the drugs for euphoria instead. Opioid-induced euphoria is the feeling of intense excitement and giddiness that some people call feeling high or getting a rush.

Perspectives on addiction and OUD vary by background and professional training. People's backgrounds tend to shape how the disorder, its treatment and root causes are viewed. For example:

- In the **mental health field**, addiction is often viewed as a psychological disorder best addressed with counseling and management of life stressors.
- Within the **legal world**, addiction may be a conduct disorder best dealt with by isolating people who take drugs from society and rehabilitating them through the penal system.
- From a **religious perspective**, addiction may be a spiritual deficiency best managed by restoring inner peace, dealing with hurt and shame and connecting to a higher power.

- From a **community's point of view**, addiction may be the natural outcome of declining social infrastructure, inadequate funding and failure to enforce policy.

What do each of these perspectives have in common? In each case of addiction, manifestations of the disorder are uniquely woven and interconnected like individual threads in a large tapestry. Every tapestry looks different because some threads are more prominent than others in creating the picture. When it comes to treatment, all are relevant and important to address.

However, there's something key missing from each of these viewpoints. Although these may help identify the who, when and where of addiction, they don't adequately address the *why* or *how*.

For instance, why can two people have the same history of personal trauma and exposure to opioids, yet only one of them develops OUD? Likewise, two people with similar spiritual practices or criminal backgrounds may have very different outcomes after trying the same type and dose of opioids.

Why do people have such dramatically different experiences with opioids? To understand the true driver of OUD, it helps to understand the science of the brain.

THE SOURCE OF ADDICTION: THE BRAIN

The human brain is built to adapt. The more people are exposed to addictive substances, the more their brains change.

> People become desperate and they become despondent. They'll do anything to support their drug habits. It's disheartening. Most people never see or even imagine the things that law enforcement sees.

PATRICK D. MCGOWAN, MINNEAPOLIS POLICE DEPARTMENT (RET.), MINNESOTA STATE SENATOR (RET.) AND HENNEPIN COUNTY SHERIFF (RET.)

Use of addictive substances like opioids alter important brain areas associated with feeling good (reward), decision-making, memory, stress and the ongoing desire to use the substance (motivation).

OUD develops as these brain areas related to pleasure, memory, decision-making and other functions change their structure and chemical pathways with repeated exposure to the drug. Looking at OUD from a thousand-foot perspective, you can see it is all interconnected by the structural and chemical changes in the brain.

The brain's biological build

Specially "hard-wired" to feel, process and respond, the brain is marvelously tuned all the way down to the cellular level to provide specific coordinated functions within each region it regulates.

Although its general appearance suggests nothing more than a bowl of linguini noodles, it's actually a highly structured and compartmentalized computer super-system with almost as many nerve connections as there are stars in the Milky Way. It has a nerve network spanning the same distance as from the earth to the moon.

When it comes to addiction, these are the parts of the brain that play key roles.

Motivation and pleasure centers

The mesolimbic pathway in the brain connects areas closely linked with a person's motivation to experience pleasure. This pathway is also known as the reward circuit. The reward circuit is activated when you do things that make you feel good, such as eat your favorite food, play a game or spend time with friends.

With repeated drug exposure, the brain develops a tolerance to the drug and the feel-good reward associated with use of the same dose diminishes. This leads the person using the drug to use higher doses or change to more potent opioids to get the same feel-good effects. With the repeated overactivation of the reward circuit, the brain undergoes changes that result in experiencing less pleasure from everyday pleasurable activities. As a result, the person becomes more dependent on a drug to experience positive sensations.

Stress and anxiety center

A part of the brain known as the amygdala contributes to feelings of stress, unease, anxiety and agitation. The amygdala is designed to let other areas of the brain know there's cause to be worried or afraid.

The amygdala plays a strong role during the addiction and withdrawal process. Withdrawal is naturally painful and distressing. The amygdala heightens the withdrawal response by making someone more anxious and uncomfortable. As a result, the person is more motivated to use the drug to avoid discomfort.

Health care providers believe the amygdala also plays a role in promoting cravings long after the last use. Because of the amygdala, people with OUD continue to use opioids, or relapse after not using them, to avoid unpleasant sensations.

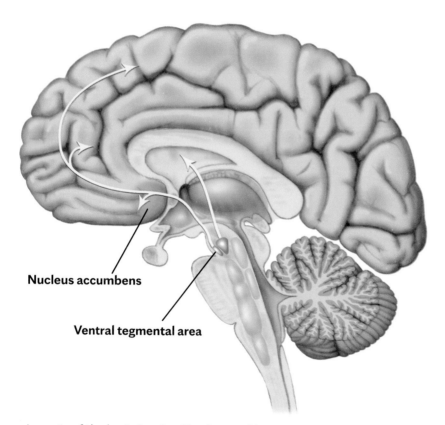

Nucleus accumbens

Ventral tegmental area

The two main parts of the brain involved in pleasurable sensations include the nucleus accumbens and the ventral tegmental area. The arrows show the flow of dopamine in the brain through the reward circuit when someone experiences pleasure.

Prioritization center

An area of the brain called the orbitofrontal cortex functions as the brain's prioritization center. It communicates with other parts of the brain to identify salience. Salience is how important something should be. Recurrent opioid use impacts the orbitofrontal cortex, and it begins to prioritize drug use over other things the person once valued, such as family, friends, hobbies and jobs.

Decision-making, problem-solving and self-control center

The prefrontal cortex is an important region of the brain dedicated to planning, problem-solving, decision-making and self-control. Repeated exposure to opioids leaves this brain region with less and less ability to regulate other parts of the brain. Such changes can lead to compulsive use of a substance, with little thought of consequences.

This area fully develops when someone is in early adulthood. Exposure to substance use during childhood and adolescence can affect brain development and how this area of the brain matures. Early substance use can result in poor impulse control and little self-regulation, with a potentially lifelong impact.

The chemicals in the mix

Nerve cells in different brain regions communicate by releasing specific chemicals called neurotransmitters. Two important neurotransmitters involved in opioid addiction include dopamine and serotonin.

Dopamine pathways impact:
• Reward (motivation).
• Pleasure and euphoria.
• Motor function.
• Perseveration, which is the continuation of an experience without stimulus.

When opioids bind to receptors in the brain, dopamine is released. Depending on what part of the brain it's released from, dopamine can control many brain functions, including movement, compulsion and repetitive activities. When it comes to addiction, it serves as the pleasure chemical.

The amount of dopamine released with opioid use differs by the route, type and amount of opioid used, along with the unique biology of the person using it. People using opioids can describe a range of sensations from no pleasure at all to full-blown euphoria. Studies show that people who experience these intense pleasurable sensations are more likely to develop addiction.

Serotonin pathways impact:
• Mood.
• Memory processing.
• Sleep.
• Cognition.

Similarly, serotonin pathways affect how "normal" you feel by regulating key activities, such as mood, sleep, memory processing and cognition. Chronic use of opioids distorts the serotonin pathway, keeping the person in a constant state of discomfort, unease and feeling generally unwell.

BECOMING IMPRISONED: A LIFE CYCLE OF ADDICTION

Each area of the brain is under constant regulation by other areas of the brain to prevent too much or too little activity. This includes the pleasure center.

Imagine if typically pleasurable activities became all-consuming and uncontrollable. Walks can be pleasurable, but few people could handle 30 miles of walking a day. A bowl of ice cream is a special treat, but you would be wider than you are tall if you made it a dietary staple.

With continued opioid use, this intricate balance of brain regulation gradually becomes distorted. A person using opioids has less and less control over behaviors. When drug use becomes compulsive and difficult to control, addiction can develop.

The life cycle of addiction evolves over time as the person taking the drugs transitions from one state to another. There are three states in this cycle:

1. The first state is **controlled use**, wherein pleasure is the primary motivator for drug use.

2. The second state is **impulsive use**, wherein someone uses the drug without thinking through the consequences of doing so as the brain starts to undergo major changes.

3. The third state is **compulsive use**, wherein preventing negative side effects of withdrawal becomes the primary driver of continued drug use.

In the beginning

Early in the cycle of addiction, the primary driver for opioid use is the pleasurable response the drug brings. People are able to control their drug use at this stage and are still able to focus on other activities.

Later in the cycle, with recurrent use, chemical and structural changes start to take place in the brain when it's exposed to opioids. More and more dopamine is released in the pleasure centers of the brain. Moderate doses of morphine, for example, increase typical dopamine levels by 100% to 200%.

This persistent surge of above-normal levels of dopamine requires that more

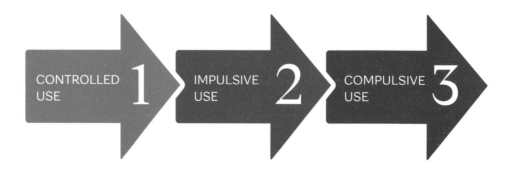

CONTROLLED USE **1** — IMPULSIVE USE **2** — COMPULSIVE USE **3**

dopamine receptors become available to handle the volume. As drug use continues over time, brain connections between the reward, memory or decision-making areas become distorted. As a result, the brain receives distorted messages about how pleasurable the next drug use activity will be.

The brain also becomes stimulated by certain triggers, such as drug-related images and sounds. These could be the sight of a needle or the creak of a door in the room where drugs are used. For some people, this transition to being triggered can occur as soon as a few weeks after starting the drug.

These changes in brain structure and function can be so powerful that nondrug triggers have been shown to activate chemical release in the same parts of the brain as the drugs themselves, acting as potential causes for relapse in people recovering from OUD.

As the brain begins to rewire, the mental processes that drive opioid use become more automatic and more efficient. Certain behaviors associated with drug use may become more prominent as the brain becomes increasingly dependent on drug-driven dopamine surges to achieve a positive mood. These behaviors may include secrecy, manipulation, excessive irritability and many other troublesome behaviors.

As drug use continues

As opioid use becomes chronic — typically defined as taking opioids on a near-daily basis for 45 to 90 days — additional brain restructuring takes place.

As the brain tries to keep up with the increased levels of dopamine and serotonin constantly flooding various areas, dopamine binding areas begin to burn out, leaving fewer receptors available for dopamine to bind to.

DOPAMINE RELEASE IN OPIOID ADDICTION

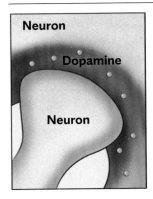

Dopamine released during normal pleasurable activities

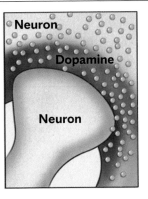

Dopamine released when taking opioids

A representation of connections in the brain of someone who is not addicted to opioids

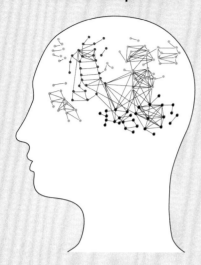

A representation of connections in the brain of someone who is addicted to opioids

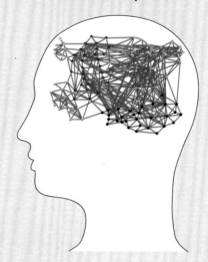

Studies have shown significant changes in brain connections in someone who is addicted to opioids.

The illustration on the left represents the brain of someone who is not addicted to opioids.

The illustration on the right represents the long-term impact on the brain of someone who is addicted to opioids.

Each colored dot represents a unique area of the brain that regulates specific activities related to drug seeking, such as motivation and decision-making. The lines between the colored dots represent connections between areas of the brain which, outside of drug use, may normally communicate very little.

When you compare the two illustrations, you can see significantly more connections in the brain of the person who is addicted.

These connections continue to exist even when the person is not using drugs.

These new or strengthened connections reduce a person's inhibition as well as affect memory and values. All these result in a greater motivation to seek drugs. These changes in the brain can last years beyond the point someone no longer uses drugs.

Pleasurable activities that lead to normal levels of dopamine release, such as hugging a family member or walking along a beach, now have less positive impact. When routine activities fail to provide pleasure, the person becomes increasingly dependent on the drug to feel happiness.

The opioid-impacted brain also rewires connections between different parts of the brain not previously well connected.

As a result, connections that were like dirt roads and side streets morph into freeways and highways. These changes make it hard for the inhibitory control centers of the brain — the parts of the brain that help you make reasonable choices and use good judgment — to override the desire to use drugs. The desire to use drugs becomes more impulsive. This means a person spends less time thinking about the risks of drug use prior to engaging in it.

THE THREE MAIN ACTIVITIES THAT DRIVE THE CYCLE OF ADDICTION

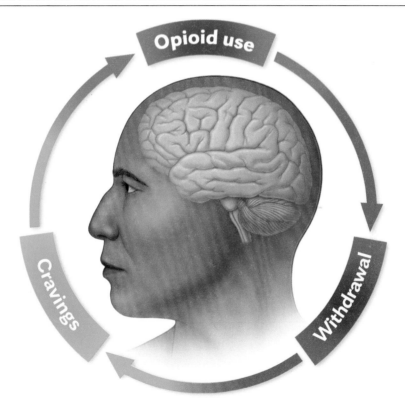

Use of opioids results in withdrawal as the drug wears off. This withdrawal drives cravings to use the drug again. The cravings result in repeated drug use, which perpetuates the cycle.

With the brain now more dependent on opioids to maintain function, withdrawal symptoms begin to emerge when the drugs wear off. Unpleasurable sensations develop within hours of no longer taking an opioid. These may include:

- Sweating.
- Restlessness.
- Stomach cramps.
- Diarrhea.
- Anxiety.
- Bone and joint aches.
- Fast heart rate.

The combination of all these changes results in a persistent state of craving, fear, anxiety and avoidance of withdrawal. At this stage, drug use becomes compulsive. This means that the need to take drugs exceeds a person's self-control system, resulting in the characteristic behaviors and patterns of use so often seen in OUD.

To make matters worse, the parts of the brain responsible for making decisions about seeking treatment don't function properly. The person is less likely to seek help and the cycle spirals out of control.

DAWN: "A HORRIBLE LIFE"

I used opioids for 15 years. I started on hydrocodone. When I was high, I'd be coloring and humming and talking nonsense. I'd drive with my kids in the car and fall asleep.

I couldn't function without pills and I couldn't keep a job. My life was all about how I was going to get my next fix. From the time I woke up until the time I went to bed, all I thought about was drugs and getting more.

I would purposely hurt myself so I could go to the hospital in pain and get pills. One time, I hit my hand with a hammer so I could go to the hospital and get drugs for the pain.

That was a horrible life.

Then I went to a doctor for two years who gave me anything I wanted. I think he got in trouble for giving too many pills, so he gave me fentanyl patches instead.

Then I overdosed on fentanyl patches. I ate one. At the hospital, they gave me seven shots of naloxone within a three-hour period. I hated the way the naloxone made me feel. Made me sick to my stomach. But afterwards, I was glad they gave it to me because it saved me.

My son was there at the hospital that day. He was 17. I put that kid through so much. He said that was the worst experience of his life. That's when I decided I wasn't touching drugs again.

Loved ones watching someone with OUD at this stage may see behaviors ranging from engaging in criminal activity to afford drug habits to the inability to hold a steady job and dealing with homelessness, withdrawing from friends and family due to shame, and struggling with depression and anxiety.

The person is trapped physically, psychologically, spiritually and socially in the prison of OUD.

WHAT DOES OUD LOOK LIKE?

Opioid use disorder may not be as obvious as you think. Because there are many roads that lead to developing OUD, the condition can take on different appearances.

Early stages may be subtle and challenging to notice. Consider the following examples:
- A health care provider may suspect OUD due to a person's reluctance to taper opioids despite the fact they're not improving daily functioning.
- Friends and family may suspect addiction because a relative or friend is irritable, secretive and shows no interest in their usual activities. The person may no longer fulfill normal obligations or responsibilities.

However, people with OUD frequently show common, recognizable signs. These include:
- Regularly taking an opioid in a way not intended by the prescriber, including taking more than the prescribed dose or taking the drug for the way it makes a person feel.
- Sleep changes, such as sleeping a lot more than usual or a lot less than usual.
- Taking opioids "just in case," even when not in pain, or taking higher doses than recommended.
- Having mood changes, including excessive swings from elation to hostility.
- Borrowing medication from other people or "losing" medications so that more prescriptions must be written.
- Seeking the same prescription from multiple doctors to have a "backup" supply.
- Making poor decisions, including putting themselves and others in danger.
- Being involved in criminal activity.
- Being involved in motor vehicle accidents.
- Showing signs of decreased academic or work performance.
- Having troubled relationships.

No matter how OUD manifests, a diagnosis is made the same way. The Diagnostic and Statistical Manual of Mental Health Disorders (DSM-5) outlines the criteria providers should use to diagnose OUD. The criteria include:
- Taking more of an opioid than intended.
- Failed attempts to stop taking opioids.
- Excessive time spent obtaining opioids.
- Cravings for opioids.
- Failure to fulfill obligations.
- Repetitive interpersonal conflicts.
- Giving up important things for opioids.
- Using opioids in dangerous situations.
- Using opioids despite knowing they are causing significant emotional or physical consequences.
- Presence of tolerance and withdrawal symptoms.

The DMS-5 questions separate OUD into mild, moderate and severe criteria, depending on the number of signs and symptoms. Criteria focus on two types of addiction signs:

- Physiological components, such as tolerance, withdrawal and cravings. Cravings are the powerful desire to use opioids.
- Psychosocial components, such as failure to fulfill obligations; interpersonal conflicts; and prioritizing drugs over personal safety, wellness, family and friends.

WHO'S AT RISK FOR OUD?

Anyone can become addicted to opioids.

Knowing this, wouldn't it be amazing to be able to analyze a drop of blood and give people their percentage risk of developing OUD? Although risk-score calculators exist, the reality is that OUD can develop in anyone at just about any time when opioids are used.

Many people with OUD have experienced such intense pleasure after using an opioid, they say they've developed addictive traits after just a few days of use. Others say they didn't develop symptoms until they had taken the drugs for weeks.

The unfortunate reality is that risk factors often aren't a reliable way to make predictions. Many people who have risk factors take opioids and never develop OUD. And people with no risk factors develop the disorder.

Medical researchers have studied exact rates of addiction resulting from opioids, but the results have varied widely. One of the largest studies on this topic found that between 3% and 19% of people using prescription opioids develop an addiction to them.

Another study found evidence of opioid misuse in almost 6% of people who received opioids for minor surgical procedures. In pain clinic studies, up to 14% of people with chronic pain were ultimately diagnosed with OUD. Some studies also found that concerning behaviors, such as faking urine drug tests and violating opioid treatment agreements, occur in almost 40% of people with chronic pain.

Another large national survey of adults in the U.S. found that around 12% of those surveyed reported misusing opioids. Of those, more than half reported using opioids without a prescription and 40% got opioids for free from friends or relatives who had opioid prescriptions.

With most national statistics hovering between an 8% to 20% chance of misusing opioids, what determines why some people develop OUD while others don't? As you'll learn, nature, nurture and drug nuances all come into play.

DRUG FACTORS

What increases the addictive potential of an opioid? When it comes to OUD, the characteristics of the opioid are one of the biggest contributors to developing the disorder. So is the length of time you take it.

High potency

In general, more potent opioids — a small amount of the drug causes a significant effect — are more likely to lead to addiction.

High doses

Taking higher doses of opioids has been linked to OUD. Higher doses have been shown to increase the risk of complications by two to three times that of lower doses.

Quick routes

The route by which an opioid is taken contributes to increased risk of developing OUD. Opioids that take longer to make it from their site of intake to the central nervous system will have less of an addictive impact than those that make it to the brain quickly, such as by injecting and snorting.

Prolonged use

Taking opioids for an extended period is one of the greatest predictors of opioid addiction. One of the largest studies in the U.S. found that, when surveyed, 26% of people receiving long-term opioids ultimately met criteria for opioid dependency within the previous year. More recent data has shown that even short-term prescriptions pose risks of long-term use (see page 53). When a provider prescribes a second (refill) opioid prescription, this doubles the risk that the person will still be using opioids a year later.

These findings highlight the incredible importance of using the right opioid, in the right person, for the right reason, in the right form, at the right dose and for the right length of treatment.

INDIVIDUAL FACTORS

In addition to characteristics related to the drugs themselves, individual risk factors have been linked to an increased risk of developing OUD.

Age

Although a person of any age can develop OUD, younger people, typically ages 18 to 45, are more likely to develop the disorder. More men than women develop OUD, although rates of female opioid abuse are rising. Other factors — such as unemployment, divorce, low levels of education and poor socioeconomic circumstances — can also increase the risk.

Genetics

Genetics play an important role. Roughly 40% to 60% of people at risk of addiction may have genetic susceptibilities. Many of these predisposing genes are tied to the risk of developing mental health conditions, such as depression, bipolar disorder and schizophrenia, which in themselves put a person at increased risk of developing OUD.

Other genetic associations are often complex links between someone's environment and gene adaptations over time. Through a process called epigenetics, environmental factors can induce long-term changes in how a gene ultimately functions. These environmental factors include traumatic experiences, drug access and stress. Epigenetics can greatly affect how someone responds and adapts to opioid use.

History of substance use disorder

Data suggests the strongest risk factor for OUD is a personal history of substance use. This includes any history of addiction to the following:
- Legal substances, such as alcohol, tobacco and medical marijuana.
- Prescribed medications, such as benzodiazepines and muscle relaxants.
- Illegal substances, such as cocaine, methamphetamine and heroin.

Some data suggest that opioid abuse rates in people with substance abuse histories are up to four times higher than in people without this history.

Family history plays an important role too, particularly if a relative with a history of addiction is a parent or full sibling. Many of these inherited associations are tied to mental health disorders that can run in families.

Depression and other mental health disorders

Mental health disorders are very common in people with OUD. In fact, between 40% and 50% of people with OUD have a reported history of a mental health disorder. These disorders include depression, anxiety, post-traumatic stress disorder, bipolar disorder, schizophrenia, personality disorders and others. Mental health disorders can both contribute to OUD or be the result of OUD.

They're also more likely to continue taking them despite lower pain scores and higher levels of function. People with depression have also been shown to have higher rates of nonmedical use and prescription misuse of opioids.

Know that mental health conditions aren't necessarily the cause of addiction. In fact, sometimes they're the result of it as chemical and structural changes take place in the brain.

People with depression are twice as likely to transition to chronic use of opioids when started on opioids for pain.

Environment

The living environment that a person is raised in has a large impact on risk of developing OUD. Exposure to substance use in the household and factors like drug availability, limited resources, poor parental support, early life adversity and trauma can all increase the risk of unhealthy substance use and addiction.

Unsafe opioid storage practices are a particularly important risk factor, as data show family members and friends are a common source of prescribed opioid medications. Pressure or influence from older siblings experimenting with drugs may influence substance use and outcomes in younger siblings.

Polysubstance abuse

"Polysubstance abuse" refers to using more than one drug that can be abused, such as taking opioids while also using alcohol, benzodiazepines, muscle relaxants or illegal drugs. Using multiple substances at one time greatly increases the risk of opioid use disorder.

In general, using any medications capable of reinforcing activity in pleasure centers of the brain increases the risk of opioid abuse.

Illegal use of opioids has been shown to correlate closely with abuse of other drugs. For example, 65% of people with a history of heroin use disorder also use nicotine products. In addition, 20% have a cocaine use disorder while 25% have an alcohol use disorder.

Conditions that overlap with addiction

People addicted to drugs also tend to experience:

Tolerance and withdrawal

Chronic use of several medications prescribed by health care providers can lead to tolerance and withdrawal.

"Tolerance" means that higher and higher doses are required over time to achieve the same effect of the drug. "Withdrawal" refers to negative symptoms that develop when the drug is no longer in a person's system.

Chronic opioid use often leads to both tolerance and withdrawal. They're expected side effects of the drug.

Medical coping

Medical coping is the use of a drug to alleviate emotional pain or problems

> Telling the difference between chronic pain and OUD can be challenging for even the most experienced health care provider.

from mental health disorders. It's a common reason many people begin to take opioids. In addition to creating the sensation of pleasure, opioids can be sedating and help reduce the effects of anxiety and depression early on in their use. People who experience significant life stressors or who have traumatic backgrounds often use medical coping as a way to manage their problems.

Chronic pain

As explained in Chapter 3, the controversial term "pseudoaddiction" was coined in the 1980s to describe certain behaviors in people with poorly controlled or undertreated chronic pain.

These behaviors included:
- Asking for opioid pain medications before the next dose.
- Requesting higher doses of opioids.
- Requesting specific opioid pain medications.
- Hoarding pain medications out of fear of feeling significant pain or not having effective means to relieve it.
- Claiming pain in attempts to get more pain prescriptions.

Not surprisingly, people with OUD do these same things. People with chronic pain may also experience tolerance and withdrawal. Like OUD, chronic pain is often associated with other mental health conditions, such as depression and anxiety.

For most people, opioids don't work to treat or manage chronic pain. Many people with chronic pain can be successfully transitioned from opioids to other drugs that do not have the same addiction risk.

Given the similarities and the high risks associated with opioid use for chronic pain, people taking opioids should be closely monitored through urine drug screens, pill counts and other monitoring methods.

KNOWLEDGE IS EMPOWERING

When you understand the true roots of addiction, you can partner with your health care provider to target interventions strategically. Although opioid use disorder affects people differently, ultimately, it results in the same destructive patterns that can take away quality and longevity of life.

In the next chapter, we discuss how scientists and researchers have used their understanding of this medical disorder to develop successful treatments to address it. Combining medications with other therapies that focus on the psychological, social and spiritual aspects of life offers a good chance of recovery.

——————— **W H A T I F** ———————

instead of shaming people who have OUD, we offer compassion, understanding and a helping hand?

Management of opioid use disorder:
10
Goals, providers and tools

Few things in life are as important as freedom — freedom to make choices, freedom to think clearly, freedom to explore and enjoy life's possibilities.

For people who struggle with opioid use disorder (OUD), freedom is often replaced with bondage — to cravings, withdrawal and social stigma. Addressing addiction involves more than just setting people free from drug use. It also means giving them back their physical health, improving their personal relationships, helping them function better at work and in society and reducing social impacts like criminal activity.

The reality is that when OUD is treated in one person, everyone benefits.

No single treatment works for all people with OUD. However, for most, a unique plan that includes medications combined with behavioral treatments offers the best chance at recovery.

In this chapter, we explore the various treatment options available for OUD and discuss how these can open the door to a better life for people using opioids and the people around them.

THE ULTIMATE GOAL OF TREATMENT

Imagine a chessboard set in front of you. The pieces are arranged, and your opponent has offered you the first move. But if this is the first time you have played chess, you're likely to ask, "What's the goal of the game?"

When it comes to OUD, you have to ask a similar question: "What is the goal of treatment?"

Historically, eliminating drug use was thought to be the right answer. But like other chronic conditions, OUD often involves going back and forth between periods of not using drugs, called sobriety, to periods of using again, called relapse.

Unfortunately, while years of research have found some effective treatments, addiction has no guaranteed cure. The combination of brain rewiring, chemical changes and long-term social challenges leaves many people at risk for relapse even after prolonged periods of sobriety.

For many who struggle with OUD, relapse will be the norm, not the exception. This is especially true for people who are addicted to more than just opioids, such as alcohol or tobacco.

Recognizing this allows the focus of treatment to move from the drug to the person. So instead of trying to completely cure addiction, the goal becomes multi-pronged: to reduce symptoms, achieve sobriety, promote recovery and improve the quality and longevity of life. These are achievable goals.

Most people with OUD begin the early part of treatment by achieving sobriety. Sobriety means no longer taking the drug in unhealthy ways. As treatment continues, they progress

The goals of treatment are to reduce symptoms, achieve sobriety, promote recovery and improve the quality and longevity of life.

to a state of recovery. This means opioid use is no longer impairing their ability to perform day-to-day functions — working, engaging in hobbies and maintaining relationships.

THE BENEFITS OF SUSTAINED RECOVERY

Sustained recovery is the end goal for everyone with OUD. Its benefits can be seen in many areas, including those listed here.

Improved personal health

During sustained recovery, people are less likely to have serious problems and complications caused by risky behaviors that are part of drug use. They're at much lower risk of:
- Acquiring illnesses from sharing needles and injecting drugs.
- Developing medical conditions from using drugs in unapproved forms, such as inhaling or snorting.
- Becoming ill from drug contaminants.
- Developing immune suppression from chronic drug use.
- Living with violence, poverty and homelessness.
- Getting poor nutrition.

Restored relationships

Chronic use of opioids often leads the people taking them to prioritize getting drugs ahead of all else, including relationships with family and friends. In recovery, relationships can be restored and ultimately these relationships can play an important role in helping sustain long-term recovery.

Better life choices

Addiction often makes people place the pursuit of drugs ahead of everything else, including holding down a job. To afford drugs, some people turn to criminal activities. In recovery, people usually do not engage in criminal activities. Studies have shown that for every $1 spent on addiction treatment, $7 are saved in criminal justice and law enforcement costs.

DIANA: "IT DOESN'T DISCRIMINATE"

I am a 54-year-old woman. I have been sober for 10 years, but I am still an alcoholic. My whole family struggles with addiction.

My son became addicted to drugs and alcohol in high school. For many years, he was deep into drugs. He was doing heroin by IV.

He was really lost for a long time. He was in and out of jail, breaking the law. He stole a car and was in a high-speed chase. He assaulted someone. This wasn't my son. This just wasn't my son.

He overdosed twice. He said he died and they brought him back. One time, he was found in a car slumped over. I don't know how many times they had to give him naloxone. It was shocking to me because I had never experienced anything like that.

He finally went through a wonderful treatment program and he is now three and a half years sober. That was his fourth time in treatment and that was the one that really stuck. His life is completely changed. I am just so grateful every day when I can talk to him and look at him.

I have a daughter who has addiction too. Her kids were taken away at one time, but she is sober now and has her kids back.

I am here in treatment now myself because I am trying to get better from addiction too.

Addiction — it's a taker; it doesn't discriminate.

I am just grateful that my kids are on the same sobriety path that I am. I just want to get better. I have my kids and my grandchildren. I want us all to be happy and healthy and sober together.

WHAT IF SOMEONE ISN'T READY FOR TREATMENT?

The decision to enter treatment often isn't an easy one. Some people need to feel they've hit rock bottom or have lost everything before they're able to accept that it's time to make a change.

It's not uncommon for people addicted to opioids to resist treatment. They may be thinking:
- "My addiction isn't really that bad."
- "I can get off the drugs myself without help."
- "Using drugs isn't keeping me from working or affecting my marriage. Why do I need to quit?"
- "It's too much work to get into treatment."
- "I've tried treatment before, and it didn't work. Why should I try again?"

The most important reason to get treatment is because addiction just keeps taking. It starts with consuming time and money. But eventually, it steals reputations, relationships, jobs, health — and for too many people, their lives.

You don't have to wait until addiction takes everything from you before you get treatment. In fact, early treatment can keep you from losing everything.

If others are concerned about your opioid use but you don't think you are ready for treatment, try it anyway. Studies have shown that people who enter treatment reluctantly achieve sobriety almost as often as those who enter treatment fully committed.

THE PATH TO GETTING HELP

Like tackling any problem in life, you have to start somewhere. People decide to seek treatment for OUD for different reasons.

Some people recognize they have a problem with drug use. This greatly increases the chance they will explore treatments. Other people end up receiving treatment because they were encouraged to do so by friends and family or because they were ordered to by the court system.

There's usually a common series of steps involved to help determine which treatment plan will most likely be effective.

The American Society of Addiction Medicine (ASAM) has developed a comprehensive assessment plan that reviews factors or dimensions that impact people, such as their medical and emotional states, whether they're actively intoxicated, their willingness to engage in treatment and life problems that could contribute to relapse.

Most often, health care providers or mental health professionals complete the ASAM assessment on page 125. It can also be performed by treatment program staff at the time someone joins a program — a process referred to as intake.

The ASAM's criteria evaluates people for six dimensions. The health care team then uses the information learned from this multidimensional assessment to create a treatment plan.

ASAM ASSESSMENT

Dimension	Questions to explore
1. Acute intoxication and withdrawal potential	What are the person's past and current experiences with substance abuse and withdrawal? Is the person addicted to other substances in addition to opioids?
2. Biomedical conditions and complications	What is the person's health history? What is his or her current physical condition?
3. Emotional, behavioral or cognitive conditions and complications	What is the person thinking and feeling? What mental health issues does the person have?
4. Readiness to change	Is the person ready to make a change?
5. Relapse, continued use or continued problem potential	Has the person been in treatment before? What are the person's risk factors for relapsing after treatment?
6. Recovery and living environment	What is the person's current living situation? What other factors in his or her life, such as friends and work, will affect recovery?

Determining OUD severity

Mental health professionals grade OUD as mild, moderate or severe by using The Diagnostic and Statistical Manual of Mental Health Disorders (DSM-5) scoring system. (You can read more about this system in Chapter 9.)

The DSM-5 score can help providers determine the type of medications, behavioral therapies and length of treatments that may be needed for a sustainable recovery.

It's important to assess whether someone is addicted only to opioids or is addicted to other substances as well, such as alcohol or other drugs. People who are addicted to more than one substance usually need different treatment plans than those addicted only to opioids.

Screening for mental illness

Part of the initial intake process often involves comprehensive screening for mental health disorders. Health care professionals screen for depression, anxiety, bipolar disorder, schizophrenia, post-traumatic stress disorder (PTSD) and other mental illnesses.

If left untreated, mental health disorders have been shown to affect treatment outcomes. If the health care team identifies that someone has a mental health disorder, the team can make a referral to the right specialists. These specialists can provide counseling and medications to manage the disorder. Addressing underlying mental health conditions greatly improves success of treatment for OUD.

For some people, addressing mental health disorders is enough to help achieve recovery from OUD. For others, the mental health disorder is determined to be the result of, not the cause of, OUD. Treatments then target OUD as the source.

THE OUD TREATMENT TEAM

Many different types of health care professionals can help someone with OUD on their recovery journey. These may include:
- Primary care physicians.
- Psychiatrists.
- Addiction medicine specialists.
- Psychologists.
- Clinical social workers.
- Nurse practitioners.
- Physician assistants.
- Counselors, including chemical dependency counselors and family counselors.
- Other program staff.

Most often, the specialists work together as a treatment team. Each member is trained to address a specific aspect of OUD. Some specialists focus on making sure the diagnosis is correct. They determine whether someone has other mental or physical health conditions that could affect recovery.

Other team members may focus on developing treatment plans, then adjusting the plans based on the progress made during treatment. Some may work with friends and community and legal support systems to help with the transition back into society.

These health care professionals can offer valuable support and play an important role in both the diagnosis and treatment of addiction. They can complete a full medical assessment to look for complications related to opioid abuse. They can also help engage family, determine a person's readiness to change, prescribe helpful medications and make referrals to treatment programs. They can connect people to community resources, such as housing and transportation. They can also help with insurance issues.

MANAGEMENT OF OUD

Ask anyone addicted to opioids what part of their life has been impacted by addiction and they'll likely respond, "All of it." For many, to be addicted is to be trapped emotionally, physically, socially and spiritually.

Escaping the grip of hijacked brain circuitry and its impact on life is challenging. For this reason, many of the most successful treatment programs use a biopsychosocial-spiritual approach to tackle OUD, in which physical, psychological, social and spiritual problems are all addressed.

Several approaches may be used to help people with OUD achieve recovery.

Biological approach

Medications serve as the biological treatment in the biopsychosocial-spiritual model and are used to support mental and physical health during treatment.

MOUD

Medications for OUD (MOUD) is the first-line treatment for most people with moderate to severe OUD. This is also known as medication-assisted treatment (MAT).

Medication treatments include certain types of approved opioids. You're likely asking yourself, "How can the source of the problem — opioids — be the answer to the problem?"

In some respects, it sounds like a cardiologist telling someone who's just had a heart attack that their treatment will involve eating two donuts every day, provided they only eat the donuts prescribed to them. If you just had a heart attack and you were told this, you would be skeptical, and rightly so!

But the principle is surprisingly sound. It's based on a deep understanding of the scientific properties of opioids and how they drive addiction.

The three FDA-approved MOUD drugs are:
1. Methadone.
2. Buprenorphine.
3. Naltrexone.

Each of these medications works in a different way. And each of these drugs allows the brain time to heal from the devastating consequences of extraordinarily high levels of neurotransmitters associated with opioid abuse.

Numerous studies show these three medications offer the most successful and long-lasting effects of the therapies currently available for OUD.

When included in the treatment plan, they can help reduce withdrawal symptoms and cravings, reduce the risk of death from overdose and improve the ability to perform day-to-day functions, called activities of daily living.

They can also improve the ability to:
- Restore relationships.
- Rejoin society.
- Function at work.
- Improve treatment engagement and retention.
- Reduce medical complications, such as infections with HIV or hepatitis C.
- Reduce the level of engagement in illegal activities.

Given these potential benefits, it's no surprise they're the first-line treatment when it comes to moderate to severe OUD.

Methadone

Methadone is the first and oldest medication used as a treatment for OUD. First developed during World War II as an alternative to morphine, its real potential was realized in the 1960s, when inner cities across America were plagued by heroin addiction.

Scientists recognized that methadone had some unique properties. Like other opioids used for pain and addiction, methadone binds to opioid receptors.

When methadone binds to the receptor, it works very slowly, which limits the euphoric sensations of dopamine release. In addition, it binds to receptors for much longer periods than many opioids, limiting withdrawal symptoms for 24 to 36 hours.

Researchers found that by using methadone for people addicted to heroin, many people were able to return to their normal lifestyles. Although people taking methadone were technically still using opioids, they could control their use.

Data suggests that people taking methadone as part of a treatment program are four times more likely to stay in treatment. And many follow-up studies have shown additional benefits of methadone, including:
- Up to a 70% reduction in death rates.
- Lower rates of HIV and other infections.
- Improved treatment participation.
- Lower chance of using IV drugs.
- Improved overall health.

Like any medication, the drug has the risk of complications, including dangerous heart rhythms. These risks can be safely managed with regular follow-up and close monitoring.

When used to treat OUD, methadone can only be prescribed through an Opioid Treatment Program (OTP), where the drug is provided directly to the person taking it. People in the program taking methadone are closely monitored. They're required to take part in psychosocial interventions, including counseling and 12-step participation programs such

WHAT'S AN OPIOID TREATMENT PROGRAM?

In the U.S., the use of medications for opioid use disorder (MOUD) is governed by the Certification of Opioid Treatment Programs, 42 Code of Federal Regulations (CFR) 8.

The regulations created a system to certify and officially accredit programs as Opioid Treatment Programs (OTPs), allowing them to administer and dispense FDA-approved medications.

To be certified as an OTP, the program must require people receiving MOUD to also receive counseling and other behavioral therapies, thus allowing a whole-person approach to treatment.

as Narcotics Anonymous. (Counseling and 12-step programs are explained later in this chapter.)

Like all opioids, methadone can lead to abuse and addiction. It can cause euphoria when taken in high doses or combined with other opioids. Methadone clinics manage methadone's abuse potential and safety risk through strict rules and regulations.

For the first few months of treatment, people taking methadone are typically required to attend appointments at the methadone treatment program on a regular basis.

Once people have proven they will faithfully participate in the program, they're usually eligible to take additional doses at home during the week. Throughout their treatment, people undergo supervised urine drug screening and must participate in other mental health treatments.

Buprenorphine

Buprenorphine has proven to be one of the most effective treatment strategies available for OUD. This is due to its unusual effects on opioid receptors.

As the drug encounters an opioid receptor, it binds tightly, preventing other opioids from attaching. Once bound, it activates the receptor. This results in reduced amounts of dopamine release and lowers the amount of euphoria the person feels.

The drug also has other unique properties. It can reduce anxiety levels, improve rates of sobriety and reduce accidental overdose. Its special chemical properties reduce the risk of it causing breathing difficulties, even when taken at higher doses.

Buprenorphine substantially lowers the rates of relapse in people taking it compared with those who don't take it.

One of the greatest benefits of buprenorphine is its value in keeping people engaged in other forms of treatment. Studies have found that up to 75% of people taking buprenorphine are able to remain engaged with other aspects of their treatment one year after they get started.

Of course, like any medication, buprenorphine carries the potential to be abused. By stimulating the opioid receptor, it offers reinforcing effects that help with compliance but also increase the risk for abuse. The abuse potential is theoretically lower than for traditional opioids because the drug doesn't cause high degrees of euphoria. Although it can be used with other opioids to increase the pleasure sensation, research suggests that many people who use street drugs do so to treat withdrawal symptoms.

Typically, buprenorphine is taken daily by placing it under the tongue. Newer forms combine buprenorphine with the opioid receptor blocker naloxone. This combination is the most commonly prescribed form of buprenorphine. Brand names include Suboxone and Zubsolv.

Newer ways to take buprenorphine include a version that can be implanted under the skin and another that can be injected safely.

These versions have improved the rates of people keeping to a treatment plan, called retention, and reduced risk of abuse when compared to versions taken by mouth.

Unlike methadone, buprenorphine can be prescribed by primary health care providers to patients in an office setting rather than only to those in a treatment program. In the past, health care providers had to have special training and a special license to prescribe the drug. However, in 2021, regulations changed to make it easier for health care providers to prescribe it to those who need it.

Just like methadone, combining buprenorphine with other forms of monitoring and psychosocial-spiritual interventions likely offers people with OUD the greatest chance at recovery.

Naltrexone

Unlike methadone and buprenorphine, naltrexone is an opioid antagonist. Antagonists completely block opioid receptors without activating them. The drug puts a lock on the opioid receptor so that opioids can't open the door and enter.

DR. MATT DAY: "THERE'S GOT TO BE A BETTER WAY"

I'm a family medicine health care provider in a small town in the Midwest. Years ago, I became interested in treating people for addiction.

At one time, we just didn't have a good program in primary care for managing the use of opioids long-term. I thought, "You know, there's got to be a better way." Then I heard about Suboxone from a colleague, and I did my research and then did the required DEA training.

That's where the whole process started. Suboxone became an option for people in treatment and I began treating a handful of patients.

People started showing up who were using heroin or methadone or prescription opioids. I have one patient who had a near-death experience and now he's on Suboxone. He has referred three or four people to me that he used to buy heroin with.

But you can't just give patients Suboxone and expect they won't be addicted anymore. About half my patients are actively involved in a treatment program outside of just doing MOUD.

Every visit, I ask, "Are you involved in meetings? Are you involved in a therapy program?"

Of course, I see people who don't get better. Some of them are highly motivated to make this work and some are not.

Because of this lock, if someone taking naltrexone tries to take another opioid, the other drug has little effect. Naltrexone doesn't have abuse potential since it blocks the receptor without activating it. It doesn't create a feeling of being high, so it doesn't have street value and doesn't lead to tolerance, dependence or breathing difficulties. It has the added benefit of encouraging the body to create natural opioids, called endorphins, which help a person feel better.

However, naltrexone can quickly lead to withdrawal symptoms if someone has another opioid in his or her body.

Multiple studies have shown that if taken as intended, naltrexone increases the chance of sobriety and decreases overdose risk. Unlike with buprenorphine and methadone, the person experiences no withdrawal when the drug is stopped, as long as there's no other opioid in the body. However, the absence of withdrawal symptoms and lack of euphoric effects often lead people to stop taking the medication too early.

For this reason, people who are going to take naltrexone must be highly motivated not to use opioids. Studies show that health care professionals and inmates on work release are the most likely groups to stay on naltrexone.

Although the drug can be taken daily by mouth, newer forms are now available, making it easier for people to stay on it. One form is injected once a month.

Data show success rates similar to buprenorphine in people willing to take the medication regularly for as long as recommended.

How long should someone be on MOUD?

Health care providers believe longer stretches of treatment are better than shorter ones. The length of treatment offered is often based on two things:
1. The recommendations by program providers.
2. The preferences and goals of the person with OUD.

For many people with OUD, their goal is to be off all forms of opioids completely. For people with this goal, MOUD is often prescribed for three to six months, followed by a tapering plan with close monitoring.

Some people remain on MOUD for a long time. All three medications can be given long-term. Sometimes, MOUD therapy is started using one medication. Then the person transitions to another medication once treatment goals have been achieved and the person has entered the maintenance stage. For example, some people are started on buprenorphine and after six months of sobriety are transitioned to long-term naltrexone.

The decision on when to begin MOUD treatment and which medication to use is

MOUD has shown excellent results when given at the right dose for the right amount of time. Studies comparing the effectiveness of buprenorphine, methadone and naltrexone appear to show similar results.

customized to the person receiving treatment and is reassessed on a regular basis.

Other medications used to treat opioid use disorder

Other medications have proven to be effective in helping relieve symptoms and medical conditions related to OUD. They include:

Antidepressants

Antidepressants are used to treat depressed moods that might make it more difficult to engage in treatment. Antidepressants reduce the risk for relapse and promote rebuilding relationships. They're particularly helpful for people who were experiencing depression before they began using opioids.

Antipsychotic medications

These medications may be helpful for people with severe mental health disorders. Antipsychotics can help them get to a state where they can successfully take part in treatment.

Medications to help with withdrawal symptoms

Certain drugs reduce stress hormone responses during withdrawal. Examples include clonidine and lofexidine (Lucemyra). The drugs can lessen symptoms such as heart pounding, muscle tension and nausea. They can also help people in the early stages of withdrawal as well as help reduce symptoms when transitioning from one type of MOUD to another.

Psychosocial approach

Psychosocial interventions also are important tools in OUD treatment. They help address problematic thinking patterns that have developed when someone has OUD. They also help establish new health patterns and build human connections by encouraging the use of social skills. Common psychosocial interventions include the following:

Individualized drug counseling

This type of counseling focuses on a one-on-one interaction between the person with OUD and the counselor. During counseling sessions, the two examine reasons for wanting to reduce or stop opioid use and address life areas that have been impacted by drug use, such as employment, illegal activities and family and social relationships. The goal is to create behavioral goals and develop coping strategies and tools to stop using opioids.

Group counseling

This type of counseling represents the foundation for most drug dependency treatment programs. It involves a specially trained staff member leading people in a group setting. The approach uses positive social pressure to emphasize treatment concepts and social norms to help promote drug-free lifestyles.

PREGNANCY AND OPIOIDS

Opioids can affect both fertility and pregnancy. If you take opioids and plan to get pregnant, talk with a health care provider. A provider can help you find other options for pain management, help you taper off opioids or reduce the dosage of opioids you take to levels that lessen their impact on fertility or pregnancy.

If you're pregnant and have opioid use disorder, you may worry about many things. You may not have planned this pregnancy and worry about its consequences, including concern for the health of your baby.

You may hesitate to get health care while pregnant because you fear what may happen. Or you may choose to not seek treatment for OUD while pregnant because you fear criminal prosecution or the possibility of losing your child to foster care after birth.

Understand that providers are concerned about your health and your baby's. If your OUD isn't treated, your baby could face serious health challenges and will be at higher risk of dying before birth. In addition, the child is at risk for premature birth, low birth weight and poor mental and physical health.

Opioid use during pregnancy also can result in a condition called neonatal abstinence syndrome (NAS). The condition develops after birth, when the baby no longer receives opioids through the mother's blood supply and the baby begins to go through withdrawal. Babies born with NAS are at risk for feeding challenges, breathing and sleeping problems and seizures.

The best way to help prevent complications related to OUD is to get treatment as soon as possible. Medications for opioid use disorder greatly improve the chance of having a healthy baby. Medically assisted opioid withdrawal may be an option for you as well.

It's important to understand that state and county officials may recommend removing your baby from your home if it appears you're not seeking help for addiction or if they believe the child's living conditions are unsafe.

Be aware that most state laws and programs related to OUD are meant to help you and your baby stay safe and healthy. People who make an effort to seek help for OUD are much more likely to have state decisions work in their favor. Community resources or local social service programs may provide additional support.

If you're pregnant and struggling with addiction, have an open, honest talk with your health care provider. You can expect to feel safe and be treated with respect and compassion.

Your health care provider can help you create a plan that includes the care you need. This plan can help you connect with other services and agencies in your community.

Family therapy

This counseling technique engages people with OUD and one or more family members in regular conversations about the effects of drug use on personal relationships and the family unit. The approach often helps family members improve communication, restore trust and set boundaries.

Contingency management

This technique has shown great success in reducing drug use. It involves offering rewards and other incentives for meeting goals. Goals may include attending therapy sessions, not using drugs or using medications as prescribed. Incentives can include financial rewards, opportunities to participate in events or outings that weren't allowed earlier or gaining new privileges.

Cognitive behavioral therapy

Cognitive behavioral therapy (CBT) involves either group or individual counseling sessions that help people recognize how inaccurate thoughts are affecting their behaviors. The goal is to help people change how they view a problem so, ultimately, they can change their behaviors.

Motivational enhancement therapy

Motivational enhancement therapy (MET) is one of the most commonly used counseling skills in substance abuse treatment. Rather than just providing advice, this technique guides people through thought processes that trigger the desire to change or improve behaviors. The interviewer generally asks open-ended questions designed to build trust and encourage people to reflect on their answers.

12-step programs

These are among the oldest and best-studied psychosocial interventions in treating substance use disorders. People regularly attend social-support activities and meetings in various stages of recovery. The 12 steps are a set of actions someone takes to support sobriety.

The program typically emphasizes spirituality and a reliance on a higher power to help people make changes. Some of the more commonly recognized programs include Alcoholics Anonymous (AA) and Narcotics Anonymous (NA).

Elements of effective psychotherapy

Before you begin any type of psychosocial intervention, ask your health care provider or substance abuse counselor whether the type offered is evidence-based, meaning there's research to support that it works to treat OUD.

Psychotherapy is particularly important for people who are addicted to more than just opioids and have an increased chance of relapse.

Effective, evidence-based psychotherapy typically includes:

- Treatment goals developed through good communication between you and the health care provider.
- A method for monitoring your progress during treatment.
- Opportunities to apply skills, strategies and insights beyond treatment settings.

If your health care provider or substance abuse counselor doesn't offer a type of psychotherapy that includes these elements, talk to them about other options.

To get the most out of psychotherapy:

- Make sure you feel comfortable with the health care provider giving the treatment.
- Be open and honest about everything.
- Remind yourself that this process can take time. Do not expect an instant cure.
- Stay focused on working toward your goals.
- Work to apply skills, strategies and insights between sessions.
- Give your provider feedback.
- Psychotherapy is often worth the effort to enjoy a healthier, happier life.

Spiritual approach

Spirituality can mean different things to different people. At its most basic level, it refers to a focus on the human spirit or soul. Many people believe spirituality is an important and integral part of their personal makeup. This makes spirituality an important topic to address during substance abuse treatment.

Spirituality can be challenging for professionals to incorporate into treatment. Some professionals want to lean exclusively on medical or psychological interventions consistent with their expertise and training.

Some people in treatment resist religion or spirituality because of their life experiences. However, studies show that people are more likely to achieve recovery if given the opportunity to explore the possibility of incorporating spiritual practices into their lives as part of their recovery process.

This makes sense. After all, addiction is characterized by loss, loneliness, shame, discouragement and despair. People going through treatment are usually looking for hope, purpose, connection and forgiveness. Spirituality often provides the hope that people desperately need.

Treatment programs or individual providers can encourage spiritual integration in the following ways:

- Support 12-step meeting involvement.
- Help find a supportive friend, called a sponsor.

The spirituality is what was missing from my life. I'd been in treatment many times before. I'm in a program now that includes spirituality. The spirituality component is what's keeping me sober.

D I A N A

- Encourage reading about the 12 steps and spirituality.
- Support involvement in religious or spiritual activities.
- Refer people to others who are skilled at nurturing growth and recovery.

Many clinical studies have shown benefits to incorporating spirituality into treatment. One of the best examples is the integration of a higher power into the 12-step model for alcohol abuse. Many research studies show treatment programs that integrate spirituality have better outcomes than those that don't.

Don't be afraid to ask what resources are available to support your spiritual health.

PSYCHOSOCIAL AND SPIRITUAL INTERVENTIONS

Medications used for MOUD have clear benefits when used on their own. So why include psychosocial and spiritual interventions too?

Psychosocial and spiritual interventions work in a way that is similar to how a cast works on a broken bone: They provide a protective structure to injured parts of the brain that allows the brain to heal in the right position.

While MOUD helps stabilize the cravings and withdrawals caused by opioid use, psychosocial interventions retrain the brain to manage stress tolerance, improve decision-making, build healthy social support networks and develop coping strategies. Spiritual interventions provide hope and purpose.

Retention rates in treatment programs that only include MOUD are often less than 50%. Combining treatments offers an opportunity to build support networks and coping skills that promote treatment completion and sustained recovery.

In a recent study, people who received treatment for addiction were asked what they felt most contributed to their long-term sobriety success. Most people said it was the psychotherapeutic and spiritual interventions, not the medications.

Studies have shown some differences in the value gained from combining therapies with the different types of MOUD. For example, studies comparing methadone by itself to methadone and counseling found that the combination of therapies provided a significant advantage over methadone alone.

Similarly, naltrexone success rates are higher when people using opioids are offered psychotherapies in a structured program. Buprenorphine results have been mixed with some studies failing to show a clear benefit when combined with other treatments.

SAMHSA HOTLINE

1-800-662-HELP (4357)

The Substance Abuse and Mental Health Services Administration (SAMHSA) offers health care providers comprehensive treatment recommendations about MOUD use in various health care settings. SAMHSA recommends including psychosocial and spiritual treatments as part of a comprehensive treatment plan for OUD.

EMPOWERED FOR CHANGE

Opioid use disorder is a treatable medical condition. Chances for a good outcome are improved when the right treatments are used. Treatment plans that account for a person's unique background and goals and that provide personal empowerment are generally the most likely to be successful.

In Chapter 11, you'll learn how to find and evaluate OUD treatment programs.

—————— **WHAT IF** ——————

we treat the whole person instead of the part we've decided is broken?

MANAGEMENT OF OUD IN PEOPLE WITH CHRONIC PAIN

Many people with OUD have chronic pain. Success in treating both these problems depends on whether they're being treated at the same time.

Two MOUD medications, methadone and buprenorphine, are FDA-approved to be used to treat chronic pain. People who have chronic pain and are being treated with one of these medications need to be carefully monitored, given their risks for abuse.

Because of the significant overlaps in brain rewiring between OUD and chronic pain, psychosocial treatments can be very helpful for treating both problems. Integrative and mind-body therapies may also be helpful. These may include biofeedback, yoga, tai chi and other mindfulness exercises. Many inpatient and outpatient treatment programs now have specialized programming that addresses chronic pain while also addressing OUD.

If a primary health care provider manages both OUD and chronic pain, people struggling with both can work with their provider to develop a comprehensive pain management plan.

Management of opioid use disorder: Treatment programs

11

With so many treatment options and environments available, it can be challenging to know where to begin to look for help. For most people, the world of addiction treatment is uncharted territory, leaving them with many questions, such as:

- What's the difference between inpatient and outpatient treatment?
- Does insurance cover therapy services? What if I am uninsured?
- Do I need a referral?
- Which treatment offers the best chance at recovery?
- Does treatment end when the program ends?

These are just a few of the reasons only 10% of people with opioid use disorder (OUD) pursue treatment. But remember that you don't need to navigate the road to recovery alone. Health care providers can be helpful partners when it comes to exploring the right type of care to gain freedom from OUD.

Here you'll read about how treatment specialists determine what treatment may be the most helpful, as well as the different types of substance abuse treatment environments and the differences between them.

No single treatment approach is right for everyone. This is why it's important to be informed.

HELP TAKING THE FIRST STEP

The first step of pursuing treatment can be the hardest. It's often helpful to gather as much information on the topic as possible so that you can make decisions that are right for you. Consider doing the following when researching treatment programs.

- Talk to a primary health care provider for a referral or recommendation.
- Speak with your insurance company to obtain a list of in-network providers and programs. In-network providers are more likely to be covered by insurance. Many insurance companies list in-network providers on their website. Tell your insurance company you're looking for coverage related to:
  – Addiction treatment services.
  – Mental health services.
  – Substance abuse disorder services.
  – Drug and alcohol rehabilitation programs.
- Talk to trusted family members, friends or clergy or other spiritual advisers.
- Search the internet for mental health, substance abuse and addiction treatment programs in your area.
- Check whether your place of employment has an employee assistance program (EAP) that can offer support and advice.
- If you're a student, inquire whether your school offers mental health services or referrals.

THE INITIAL ASSESSMENT

Since the effects of OUD can differ from person to person, the substance abuse treatment field offers various degrees of treatment intensity.

During an initial assessment of someone with OUD, a health care professional or mental health specialist determines the level of care the person needs. This initial assessment is often called a chemical dependency assessment.

The chemical dependency assessment has three parts:

1. **Background information.** The individual seeking treatment fills out forms pertaining to their drug use and medical and mental health history.
2. **Personal interview.** A chemical dependency assessor, usually a drug and alcohol counselor, interviews the person. The goal of the interview is to assess risk factors for addiction and severity of the addiction. This information is then used to build a treatment plan.
3. **Follow-up communication.** The assessor compiles treatment recommendations and shares them with the person seeking treatment. The information can then be shared with treatment program professionals for review.

Sometimes, insurance companies and treatment programs require a chemical dependency assessment before accepting a person into a program. Insurance coverage may also determine the length and type of treatments available.

Chemical dependency assessments are often done by staff in a treatment program. Licensed drug and alcohol counselors within the community are also often able to complete these.

Talk with the treatment program you're interested in to learn more about whether this step is completed by their program or where it can be completed within your area.

Detoxification

Detoxification, or detox, refers to medical assistance for people going through substance withdrawal. Because withdrawal is usually very difficult, people will continue to use drugs or alcohol simply to avoid the trauma of withdrawal.

Detox isn't the ideal way to begin treatment for OUD. In fact, studies have shown that up to 90% of people using heroin take the drug again after detox unless they're transitioned to medications for opioid use disorder (MOUD) therapy, such as buprenorphine, methadone or naltrexone.

Detox should always be followed by a formal chemical dependency assessment and referral to treatment.

COMMON TREATMENT ENVIRONMENTS

Treatment may occur in different settings.

In-office treatments

Buprenorphine and naltrexone are two forms of MOUD that can be offered by health care providers in a medical office setting. Providers prescribe medications to their patients for use at home.

The Substance Abuse and Mental Health Services Administration (SAMHSA) has developed guidelines for health care providers who offer MOUD, outlining methods for screening, monitoring and psychotherapy referrals.

People receiving MOUD should be referred by their provider to counseling and other behavioral intervention facilities or programs.

Outpatient treatments

With outpatient programs, participants attend appointments in a clinic setting and then go home. For people who have stable living environments and good family support, outpatient treatments are the best option.

Outpatient programs offer treatments that allow people to live in their homes and often continue to work or go to school.

There's a wide variety of types and intensities of services offered, but most outpatient programs use a group-treatment model. That means that many of the services are offered in a group environment.

Outpatient treatments can be cost-effective options because they don't include the cost-of-living expenses of an inpatient program. People receiving treatment can live with their families. This can help improve family dynamics. They can also continue to work.

Outpatient treatment isn't right for everyone, though. Sometimes outpatient treatment opens the door for relapse because it's easier for people to return to the environmental and lifestyle circumstances associated with previous drug use.

More intensive outpatient programs offer all-day treatment that can provide the same number of treatment hours as those offered at residential programs.

Inpatient programs

Your health care provider may recommend a more intensive inpatient program if you struggle socially or have more severe OUD or a history of relapse. In this type of program you live with other people in the program at a designated facility.

Inpatient — also called residential — programs provide full-time living environments, and both short-term and long-term programs are available.

Short-term programs are usually between 14 and 90 days. Long-term programs can be up to 12 to 15 months long. The length of treatment generally depends on the progress a person makes during treatment.

MODIFIED THERAPEUTIC COMMUNITIES

Long-term programs frequently use a treatment approach called a modified therapeutic community (MTC). In this program structure, people with OUD are immersed in a community environment that focuses on overall lifestyle changes to promote recovery while still receiving biopsychosocial treatments for OUD.

Those enrolled are active participants in their treatment plans and in the care of their peers. They're given more personal responsibilities as they progress through the program.

By the time people leave or graduate from the program, they're often mentally, physically and socially equipped to rejoin society with the tools necessary to avoid relapse.

Multiple studies have shown substantial benefits to using the MTC approach for people who haven't had success with other methods. MTCs have also been proven to be cost-effective given the reduced risk of relapse in comparison to short-term programs.

Residential treatment programs may provide MOUD and counseling. Many also offer psychiatric services, vocational training and other forms of psychosocial therapy.

The value of a residential treatment program is that it limits substance exposure as well as potential triggers for relapse. With structured daily routines, people receiving treatment are able to avoid distractions and focus on their rehabilitation.

Residential programs are especially helpful for people addicted to multiple drugs. Because opioids lead to changes in the brain's pleasure pathway, each abused substance reinforces the abuse of other drugs. This is a difficult cycle to stop. Residential programs often offer more intense programming designed to address this situation, known as polysubstance addiction.

Aftercare programming

After completing a treatment program, people often are asked to engage in aftercare programming. Aftercare programming helps ensure people have regular, long-term follow-up and a community support system.

Aftercare can help reintroduce someone with OUD back into society by providing relapse-prevention and support services. These services may include:
- Regular meetings or group activities.
- Pairing a person with a mentor or coach.
- Offering regular access to mental health care, MOUD and other efforts.

Many treatment programs offer their own aftercare programs. Often, people who've achieved recovery are referred to 12-step programs for ongoing support. Aftercare has proven to be an important part of care for people recovering from OUD.

ASAM PLACEMENT CRITERIA

Intensity of services

- Early interventions
- Outpatient treatments
- Intensive outpatient treatments
- Intensive outpatient
- Partial hospitalization
- Residential treatment
- Clinically managed low-intensity residential
- Clinically managed medium-intensity residential
- Medically monitored high-intensity residential/inpatient
- Medically managed intensive inpatient (hospital) treatment

Choosing the right environment

An important goal of treatment is to choose the right recovery environment for each person. To help make this key decision, many health care providers refer to the American Society of Addiction Medicine (ASAM) placement criteria.

MOUD, psychosocial and spiritual interventions also play an important role in recovery. When paired with the right treatment environment and offered for the right length of treatment, this approach has proven very effective in treating OUD.

The program you begin with may not be the one you stay with. As people with OUD progress in a chosen environment, many can be transitioned to a less intensive setting. For example, some people begin treatment in a residential program, then progress to outpatient treatment services a couple of months later.

QUESTIONS TO ASK

Remember, people with OUD have the best chance at recovery when they receive the right treatment services from the right type of providers

---

KEVIN: "YOU KNOW WHAT'S AT STAKE"

When I was in my teens, I was addicted to crack cocaine. But I got off it and was clean for six years. Then I had surgery and they gave me oxycodone for pain. In less than a month, I was addicted again.

My life got out of control. On Christmas Eve one year, I sat in my car with a gun in one hand and my phone in the other. I was about to commit suicide. I called home and I could hear my kids' voices saying, "Daddy, when are you coming home?"

I broke down crying and put the gun down. How did I get here? How on earth did I get here?

You have to think about what's important to you. How bad do you feel? How bad does your family feel? How bad are they going to feel if something really bad happens? What are you doing to the people who love you?

If something bad happens to you, you aren't going to hurt anymore — but they will.

I went into treatment. I did that to save my family. If you're addicted, go into treatment motivated by something other than yourself. You have to become selfless. Go from selfish to selfless.

You just can't go near the drugs ever again. They are just going to cause more pain. Make treatment work because you know what's at stake.

for the right length of time with the right medications.

When choosing a treatment program, consider the following questions.

Does the program offer a spectrum of environments?

Many programs offer a range of treatment environments from inpatient to outpatient to aftercare. Ask what treatment environments are available and what criteria are used to move people between treatment environments.

One benefit of selecting a program that offers a spectrum of environments is that relationships with program staff and treatment plans can often be maintained when moving from one environment to another.

In addition, medical and mental health records may not need to be transferred, and it may be easier to secure insurance coverage for a single program than making a switch partway through treatment.

Does the program offer a spectrum of services?

People with OUD often have other mental health and physical disorders. Ask which treatments are available through the program and what types of services would need to be arranged outside the program. For example, if you're depressed, ask if you'll be able to receive treatment for your depression while in the program.

Many programs have on-site psychosocial services and psychiatrists to medically address mental health disorders, such as depression and anxiety. These psychiatrists can also prescribe MOUD.

Programs that follow a biopsychosocial-spiritual approach to manage OUD typically have components that address the disorder comprehensively through a spectrum of services.

Does the program take goals into account?

Management of addiction is a partnership. People who seek treatment often come with specific goals in mind. They may include:
- Not taking opioids, including MOUD, ever again.
- Being able to see and visit their families on a regular basis for support.
- Continuing to work while receiving treatment.

Ask whether staff can help with specific goals during treatment and how these goals may impact treatment outcomes.

Does the program offer services by licensed providers?

Unlike other health care fields, mental health and substance abuse treatment programs often don't require monitoring by regulatory organizations or state health departments.

Ask whether treatment providers in the program are licensed in their respective fields. Licensed providers, such as counselors and social workers, are required to practice according to standards set by their licensing fields and to keep up with updates in their fields through regular education. Programs licensed by state health departments are typically held to certain practice standards that standardize the quality of care that should be delivered.

With nonlicensed programs, services may not be structured or delivered in a manner that meets industry standards of care.

What are the costs?

Costs for substance abuse treatment vary substantially by program — ranging from free to thousands of dollars each day. In general, programs considered not-for-profit are usually more affordable than for-profit programs.

When considering costs, request an estimate of daily, weekly and monthly service fees. Ask what types of treatments are provided for these fees. Ask about other costs, including mental health services, medical care, and room and board fees for inpatient environments.

Although costs for treatment can be significant, look at addiction services as a long-term investment. Also consider the potential money saved that otherwise would have been spent on purchasing drugs. Many treatment programs are not-for-profit, which helps lower costs.

Is the program covered by insurance?

Many programs accept insurance or government payment in the form of:
• State-financed health insurance.
• Medicaid.
• Medicare.
• Private insurance.
• Company-covered services.

To ensure expenses are covered, always check with your insurance company to be sure all proper authorizations have been obtained before enrolling in a treatment program. For more information about working with an insurance company and coverage questions, read Appendix E.

How does the program determine success?

Like many things, with OUD, outcome matters. Review each program for its rates of:
• **Program dropouts.** This is the percentage of people who leave a program before completing it.

HIPAA

The Health Insurance Portability and Accountability Act (HIPAA) prevents patient health information from being released without the patient's consent. This means that family and friends cannot be informed of a patient's treatment status or progress without the patient's consent.

- **Recovery.** This is usually defined as program participants being drug-free at least six months or one year after treatment.
- **Relapse.** This is the percentage of people in the program who relapse. To relapse is to return to drug use. This may include how often people need additional outside treatment or return to the program for repeat treatment.
- **Employment.** This is the percentage of people who return to work after treatment.
- **Criminal activity.** This is the percentage of people who engage or reengage in criminal activity after completing a program. Another term for this is the recidivism rate.
- **Overdose.** This is the percentage of program participants who overdose on opioids.
- **Client satisfaction rates.** This is the percentage of people who are pleased with the services they received in the program.

How does the program track progress during treatment?

Most programs have treatment goals based on standard definitions of program success and people's individual goals.

For some, this may involve meeting milestones set in counseling sessions or staying engaged in treatment for certain lengths of time. For others, it may be based on personal goals, such as being weaned from MOUD or having reduced opioid cravings.

When evaluating a treatment program, ask how they set and monitor goals within the program and how people can collaborate with program staff to help set personal goals.

What is the program's relapse policy?

In OUD, relapse is often the norm, not the exception. Given this, most reputable treatment programs have policies to support people through a relapse. However, some programs terminate people from treatment after relapse.

What are the program's communication policies?

More intensive programs may have policies that restrict contact with friends and family to limit distractions and potentially harmful influences. Ask what policies are in place for communicating

People who use spend 95% of their time trying to get drugs. So, when they stop, they suddenly have a ton of time on their hands. You have to fill this time. For me, it's playing the guitar. I fix guitars and I write music and I just play for myself. I go to work and I stay busy.

_____

BRAD

with friends and family while a person is in treatment and at what point during treatment these policies change.

Does the program arrange community transition and aftercare?

Data show most substance abuse relapses occur during the transition back into the community. Many programs use relapse-prevention methods, such as:

- Teaching how to reintegrate into the community after program completion.
- Preparing the family.
- Ensuring skills are in place for job placement.
- Creating a relapse-prevention action plan.
- Identifying potential relapse triggers in the home and work environments.
- Pairing with a coach or sponsor.
- Helping establish continued outpatient treatment with MOUD.
- Engaging people with support groups, such as 12-step programs.

EVERYONE IS PART OF THE TEAM

OUD is a complex condition best treated in a program that meets the unique needs of the person taking opioids. People with OUD and their friends and families should feel empowered to talk with their health care providers openly about the disorder and how to find the best treatment program for the greatest chance of success.

While health care providers play an important role in navigating the many

Over the years, I have learned things that didn't work to help me stay sober and things that did. I made conscious choices. I got rid of the phone I used to contact drug dealers. I deleted phone numbers for anyone I knew who used.

—————————————

BRAD

steps involved in treating OUD, family and friends play just as big a role. In the next section, we talk about the many ways friends and families can play an active role in preventing and managing opioid-related complications in loved ones taking these drugs.

———————— **WHAT IF** ————————

getting treatment for OUD was about more than just getting sober?

————————————————————

Helping loved ones with opioid use disorder

Opioid use disorder (OUD) is a complex medical condition that can affect virtually every aspect of someone's ability to function. These functions include personal health, relationships, work and involvement in the community.

Not surprisingly, the impact of drug abuse extends far beyond the person with OUD. The disorder can add constant chaos and instability to their lives. Friends and family often find themselves struggling to fill the roles their addicted loved one no longer can. Some rearrange their lives to support loved ones through treatment.

In this chapter, we discuss how loved ones of people struggling with OUD are impacted by the disorder and the many ways they can contribute to their loved one's recovery.

All supporters are heroes — and can serve as some of the greatest determinants of recovery success.

EARLY STAGES OF ADDICTION

Early on, addiction may only have a small impact on family dynamics. Perhaps the addicted family member doesn't show up for family events as often as before or doesn't seem to be engaged in other activities. Or maybe the person gives more abrupt or frustrated replies to questions or seems withdrawn. Maybe the person becomes more secretive or no longer fills typical roles.

These changes in a loved one can be subtle — so subtle that others may wonder whether they're happening at all. In the early stages of addiction, it's easy for friends and family to minimize concerns.

Sometimes, family members may bring up questions about certain changes but easily accept the answers provided. Other times, they're hesitant to provoke an argument and choose not to ask questions at all. And not uncommonly, families compensate by picking up the slack related to unfulfilled responsibilities.

Trust may still exist at this point, and not all family members may suspect a problem. Overall, the impact of early substance abuse on the family may be small, with only those closest to the person involved able to notice something's wrong.

JAMIE: "I HAVE A PURPOSE NOW"

I have addiction. I was an alcoholic and I did meth and I used opioids like Vicodin. I would use an opioid when I was coming off meth — anything to help me fall asleep.

Then I had teeth pulled. The doctor gave me opioids but what they gave me wasn't strong enough so I sold it so I could get something stronger. I was dating someone who was addicted to opioids so a lot of what I was doing was to get opioids for him.

I would do a "hospital hop." I'd go to a hospital and say I was in pain, and they would give me opioids. And then I'd go to another. If I wasn't selling the pills, I was using them or giving them to the guy I was dating.

My family has addiction. My mom is an alcoholic, my dad is an alcoholic, my brothers are addicts. It goes from generation to generation. My grandma is even in recovery. We don't talk about it. When something bad would happen — silence. We enable each other.

My dad is trying to be supportive of me now. He knows how hard it is to quit. He was in pain, and they wanted to give him oxycodone, but he didn't take it because he knew his limits.

I was sitting in jail for my fifth DUI. I knew I could go to prison this time. They gave me the option to go to treatment. I am in treatment now and I've been sober six months.

I have helped people here. I see other people coming in so broken and struggling and still coming off opioids. I helped someone coming off heroin. That was a good feeling. I have a purpose now.

LATER STAGES OF ADDICTION

As the person with OUD becomes more dependent on opioids to reduce withdrawal symptoms and achieve a sense of pleasure, they often engage in behaviors that begin to dismantle the family unit.

Unemployment, disability and financial difficulties create hardships that place the burden of survival on other family members. The loss of normal relationships, communication, family rituals, routines and family roles all contribute to unstable living environments. Conflict, secrecy, emotional instability and fear become the new normal.

A partner or spouse is often the first one to experience the effects of this collapse. Feelings of mistrust, neglect, loneliness, anger, blame and resentment are just a few of the emotions that can begin to surface. Good communication becomes rare. When communication does happen, it can be chaotic and hostile.

Many people don't understand how their loved one could choose a drug over family and friends. Often, a poor understanding of how addiction works drives family members to wrongly assume their loved one simply doesn't want to stop using.

Breakdown of the family unit can have particularly damaging consequences on young children and other dependent family members. Studies show that the highest rates of OUD and overdose deaths are in people ranging in age from their 20s to their 40s. These are the prime parenting years.

Reports from the U.S. Department of Health and Human Services indicate significant increases in children in need of foster care due to having parents with OUD. And, unfortunately, the consequences of addiction are often passed to the next generation. Not surprisingly, children of parents with OUD have significantly higher rates of behavioral, emotional, psychiatric and substance abuse-related issues.

FAMILIES ARE KEY TO RECOVERY

Families struggling through the chaos of having a family member with OUD may feel overwhelmed. Many may feel like they're living in survival mode.

As difficult as this is, studies show that proactive and engaged family members play an invaluable role in getting loved ones to seek treatment and supporting them throughout the recovery process.

Family members can be the primary drivers to encourage people to seek treatment. They can help restore family balance, reengage members in their respective roles and set boundaries and expectations for moving forward.

HOW TO ADDRESS OUD IN A LOVED ONE

Recognizing and confronting someone who has OUD can be daunting. But with the right tools and a plan in place, it may be the best chance to help a loved one get treatment.

The remainder of this chapter is for families and friends of those struggling with OUD. It includes information about how to recognize the disorder, compassionately address it and provide support throughout treatment.

Is opioid misuse happening in my home?

Every opioid story is different. Because of this, it may not be easy to tell whether someone is abusing opioids, especially in the early stages. Chapters 5 and 9 include

SAM: "WELCOMING ME BACK WITH OPEN ARMS"

I started using heroin when I was 18. First, I snorted it; then I injected it by IV. My dad and boyfriend were using it that way, so it was all around me. I decided I wanted to try it. That was a very bad choice.

When I would use fentanyl, I would overdose, and someone would have to give me naloxone. I can't even tell you how many times I've overdosed, probably 20 times, maybe more. I've been given naloxone many, many times.

I don't know why I kept going back to using. When I would overdose and I would come back, I would say, "Where are my drugs? Where is my heroin?"

I've had three major heart infections from the IV drug use. The first one I got when I was 21. I had a staph infection on the main heart valve. I had to be in the hospital for over a month. When I was 22, I got another infection called endocarditis* and had to be in the hospital for two weeks. When I was 23, I got MRSA** in my heart. It's amazing that I didn't have to have heart surgery or a transplant and that I didn't die.

The last time I was sitting in the hospital, the doctor was like, "You are going to kill yourself if you don't get help."

That's when I knew I needed to get treatment. When I first went into treatment, I used Suboxone. I used it for just a couple months, then I tapered off. It was really hard, but I hung in there. But my goal was to not be on any drugs at all.

I totally cut everyone out of my life at one point. But now my family supports me, I have restored relationships with them. They are welcoming me back with open arms.

I've been sober for 16 months.

"Endocarditis" is short for the condition infective endocarditis. It's a serious infection of a heart valve.

**MRSA stands for methicillin-resistant Staphylococcus aureus, commonly called "staph." MRSA is a specific type of staph bacteria that's resistant to many antibiotics. It's a common, hard-to-treat infection in people who inject drugs.*

the common risk factors that increase the likelihood of someone developing OUD.

Remember, OUD is an unpredictable disorder. People with stable home lives, solid jobs, trustworthy track records and unlikely backgrounds can easily succumb to the power of addiction.

Loved ones are the first line of defense when it comes to identifying early signs of drug abuse. It is easier to be vigilant when you know what to look for. Perhaps it's noticing changes in a loved one's moods or behaviors that don't add up.

For many, feeling that something is not quite right may be the first sign to look deeper. If you feel this way, pay attention to those concerns. Don't ignore that quiet, persistent inner voice. If your instincts are right, speaking up can help save the life of someone dear to you.

Sometimes, people outside the immediate family see the red flags. These red flags may be missed by those who are closer to the situation or who don't want to accept what's happening. This is understandable. Most people do the best they can, guided by early experiences with the person they love. Prior experience and a history of trust are two of the key reasons it can be difficult to accept that a loved one is struggling with addiction. Listen to those people who share their concerns with you.

No one wants to believe that someone they love has OUD. Knowing how to recognize opioid use disorder in loved ones is the first step.

Common signs of OUD include:
- Regularly taking an opioid in a different way than intended by the provider who prescribed it, including taking more than the prescribed dose or taking the drug for the way it makes a person feel rather than to treat a condition.
- Appearing to be high, unusually energetic or revved up, or the opposite — that is, sleepy or sedated.
- Taking opioids "just in case," even when not in pain.
- Changing moods, including excessive swings from elation to hostility.
- Borrowing medication from other people or "losing" medications so that more prescriptions are needed.
- Seeking opioids from more than one health care provider or medical facility.
- Making poor decisions, including putting themselves and others in danger.
- Being involved in crime.
- Being involved in motor vehicle accidents.
- Showing signs of decreased academic or work performance.
- Having troubled relationships.

Early in addiction, people may still go to work and take care of their other responsibilities. They may appear to maintain stability at work and home. Over time, however, the addiction is likely to lead to serious problems with their health and in all other aspects of life, such as their personal relationships, finances and lifestyle.

You may also experience changes in your own thoughts and behaviors. You may find yourself:
- Worrying about your loved one's drug use, with emotions ranging from

persistent anxiety to fear the person is going to die.

- Blaming yourself for your loved one's behavior.
- Lying or making excuses for your loved one's behavior.
- Withdrawing from your loved one to avoid mood swings and confrontations.
- Withdrawing from family and friends to prevent them from noticing what is happening.

Consider talking to your loved one's health care provider if you have concerns. The health care provider who prescribed the opioids is a key member of the care team that can help address the addiction.

Be aware of medical privacy laws. Health care providers cannot share information about your loved one's care with you unless they have received permission. However, as a family member, you can share information with health care providers about your loved one.

IF YOUR LOVED ONE IS READY FOR TREATMENT

Family and friends can play a strong role in supporting people with OUD to enter and stay in treatment.

Once your loved one with OUD expresses a willingness to enter therapy, help may be needed to explore treatment services. See Chapters 11 and 12. Different programs integrate families in different ways, so before enrolling, ask the treatment team how you can best support your loved ones through the treatment process.

For me and my family, yeah, we have things we're working through. The most important thing is we're coming together and understanding that we can get through this and grow through this.

DIANA

Following are some key steps friends and families can take while someone is getting treatment:

Stay engaged in care

To the extent allowed by the treatment program, continue to be involved in the treatment sessions, programming and social support of your loved one. Sometimes, this may involve the responsibility of monitoring the security, dispensing and taking of MOUD.

Help fill the gaps

Entering treatment may mean your loved one is no longer able to fulfill the responsibilities they previously carried. These responsibilities may include:

- Providing financial support.
- Taking care of children or pets.
- Driving family members to places they need to go.
- Preparing meals or performing household chores.

Entering treatment is the most important decision a person can make for themselves and those they love. By helping with these responsibilities, you can help your loved one focus on treatment.

Prevent access to opioids

If there are medically prescribed opioids still in the household that are being used for a legitimate, medical purpose by another family member:
- Store opioids in a locked container.
- Keep opioids in their original package.
- Do not share medication.
- Safely dispose of unused pills.

See Chapter 5 for information about safe storage and disposal of opioids.

Know the signs and symptoms of opioid overdose

Some medications used to treat OUD, such as methadone and buprenorphine, are still opioids. They can lead to life-threatening complications if not taken exactly as prescribed.

Seek emergency help if you believe someone:
- May have overdosed.
- Shows changes in consciousness.
- Has trouble breathing.

Be prepared in the event of an overdose

Whether opioids are taken as MOUD or during a relapse, be ready by:

- Keeping naloxone with you at all times.
- Asking a pharmacist or health care provider how and when to use naloxone.

RELAPSES HAPPEN — HAVE A PLAN

Unfortunately, even with OUD treatment, relapses are often the norm, not the exception.

Studies show that between 30% and 90% of people with OUD relapse. To relapse means to use an opioid again in an unsafe manner. The risk of relapse depends on many factors, including:
- The person's history of drug use.
- Types and lengths of treatments the person has received.

OUD relapse often occurs in three stages.

First, there's an emotional relapse, in which the individual experiences similar emotions to those felt when under the influence of opioids. Both happy and sad emotions can trigger an emotional relapse. Friends and family may notice the person is less engaged in conversation or just seems off.

Next, there is a mental relapse, in which the person starts to focus their thinking patterns on opioids. Thoughts may revolve around the good feelings produced while using drugs and how to access them again. This is the stage where the person begins justifying the relapse. Friends and family may notice a loved one is talking more about opioids or seems less engaged in treatment.

Finally, there's a physical relapse, which is when they use drugs again.

For many, relapse is a one-time experience and doesn't necessarily mean a permanent return to their former life of addiction. With the right social support and encouragement, many people can return to a state of sobriety quickly and may not require treatment again.

If you think your loved one has relapsed, contact his or her treatment team. Ask about next steps, including how to communicate with your loved one about the relapse.

Relapse-prevention action plans

A relapse-prevention plan is usually developed during treatment intake or later as part of treatment. These plans help people identify emotional, mental and physical behaviors that place them at risk for relapse. The plan also outlines a series of steps to take if a relapse happens.

It's your loved one's responsibility to develop this plan and put it in place. Ask whether this plan can be shared with you so you can know what to expect.

The document usually contains the following:
- A list of triggers to avoid or manage, such as:
  - Certain environments, activities or people.
  - Certain emotions, such as happiness, fear or depression.
  - High-stress situations.

- A list of behaviors that might suggest drug use, such as:
  - Talking about drugs more often.
  - Showing less interest in treatment.
  - Having mood swings ranging from depression to elation.
  - Impulsive and self-destructive activities.
  - Engaging in the same activities or socializing with the same social groups as before treatment.
- A list of prevention tools and resources to use when someone is thinking about using opioids again.
- A list of the friends, family members and clinical support team members to call if someone is thinking about using opioids again.
- A list of activities that help focus energy away from drug use. This may include exercising, journaling and engaging in family time.
- A list of support group activities like Narcotics Anonymous or other peer-support events.

TAKE CARE OF YOURSELF

Studies indicate that family members of people struggling with addiction have poor quality of life compared with those families not affected by addiction. Their stress and anxiety levels often are high. The breakdown of relationships coupled with the hardships that addiction can cause have a tremendous impact on a person's well-being.

If you have a loved one with OUD, consider these suggestions.

Learn about addiction

Understanding how addiction works can be helpful. Chapter 9 outlines how addiction develops within the brain. Understanding addiction can help explain behaviors and patterns that might not otherwise make sense to you. It can be comforting when you know others have had similar experiences.

Websites of reputable organizations, such as the Centers for Disease Control and Prevention (CDC), the National Institute on Drug Abuse (NIDA) and the Substance Abuse and Mental Health Services Administration (SAMHSA), can provide helpful information. See Appendix F for more helpful resources.

If you have a treatment program lined up, be sure to ask about family services such as community groups and online forums.

Make your own health and well-being a priority

Consider the following strategies to maintain your health and reduce stress and anxiety:
- Keep physically active. Going for just a 20-minute walk every day can be helpful.
- Engage in mind-body exercises. This includes practices such as yoga, tai chi and meditation.
- Engage in life outside your home. Consider taking up a new hobby or joining a social group, such as a book club.
- Seek spirituality. If spirituality is important to you, stay engaged in faith activities, spend time enjoying the outdoors or listen to inspirational music.
- Stay in good company. Your support journey doesn't have to be a lonely one. Having a support group with whom you can share your stories, ask questions or visit with can be lifesaving.

Consider therapy for yourself and your family

For many people living with someone struggling with addiction, the journey involves hurt, pain and betrayal. These can have a long-lasting effect on mental health, quality of life and the ability to support the addicted person through recovery.

Family and couples counseling can be critical tools to heal the mind and help process previous damages to the relationship. Individual counseling can provide an opportunity to speak openly about your feelings.

Community Reinforcement and Family Training (CRAFT) and Unilateral Family Therapy (UFT) are examples of programs meant to help family members understand addiction. The programs help family members address issues of addiction even when the loved one is in denial or refuses to get treatment.

Taking part in such programs can help families improve communication, reinforce positive attitudes toward abstinence and recovery, and learn how to recognize and prevent situations that may trigger substance use.

Interventions are often tailored to specific family needs and may focus on things such as:

- Age-specific approaches, such as for teens or older adults.
- Certain living circumstances such as military members, veterans, those who are pregnant and couples.
- Specific issues, such as parenting skills, boys' and girls' groups and big brother and big sister programs.

Consider becoming involved in a family support group, such as Nar-Anon or Narateen. Support is also available through SAMHSA's National Helpline, 1-800-662-HELP (4357).

Focus on today

It's possible that decisions you made in the past have affected the present. You may have regrets about things you've done or said. Instead of reliving the past, focus on recovery-related goals and how to get there. Your optimism and clear focus may help keep your loved one on the right path toward sobriety.

RECOVERY IS A MARATHON, NOT A SPRINT

Recovery takes time. Expect bumps in the road, unexpected turns, hills and valleys. At times, your loved one may stumble. But when someone with OUD has support, clear focus on a goal and a treatment plan, that person has a good chance of getting back up and staying on course.

——— **WHAT IF** ———

you choose to hold their hands when they lose their grip on life?

13

The intervention

Talking with someone you love about their opioid use may be one of the most difficult conversations you have in your life. But it can also be the most important.

There are times when it's clear that a loved one has a problem but isn't willing to consider treatment. This is when it may be necessary to have an intervention.

An intervention is a conversation that is carefully planned to address a harmful situation in a person's life. In the case of opioids, it addresses a person's addiction. An intervention can be initiated by friends, family, health care providers, addiction specialists or anyone with an interest in helping someone recover.

Understandably, it may seem like everything is a barrier when you try to have

this conversation. Many people have these questions:

- Is now the right time?
- Are things really that bad?
- Do they truly have an addiction? Or are their behaviors caused by something else such as uncontrolled pain?
- Should I wait until things get worse?
- What if they refuse to talk about my concerns?
- What if I'm wrong about whether they have an addiction problem?
- Will this conversation just drive them deeper into the addiction?
- Will I mess up our relationship by bringing up this topic?
- How can I avoid being too harsh or too soft?
- Can I control my own emotions?
- What if they just point out my own faults or blame me for their problems?

- Even if they want help, do I know how to provide it?

These are some of the barrier you may face. But don't let them stop you! Know that you're only responsible for speaking honestly and compassionately with the goal of getting your loved one needed help. You can't control another person's reactions.

Be prepared for your loved one to show little interest in having this conversation and to try to end it as quickly as possible. Denial, downplaying, anger, blaming, resentment, a sense of betrayal and violent displays are all common reactions.

Interventions are most likely to work when handled in an organized way. When you're aware that this type of conversation may produce highly charged emotions, you can prepare by having planned responses to help calm the conversation and keep it moving forward.

Before you talk, write down some key points about opioids and opioid use disorder (OUD). Write down what you've observed about your loved one's behavior and the actions that concern you.

Approach the conversation with facts in an honest, loving, nonjudgmental and open manner. Keep these two goals in mind:
1. To encourage your loved one to get help.
2. To ensure a safe environment for the other members of the household, now and in the future.

Understand that you may need to have several interventions over time. If your loved one cuts short the conversation, take comfort in knowing you took a small step forward. Think of each conversation as planting a seed.

BEFORE THE INTERVENTION

Plan ahead to give yourself the best chance of helping your loved one.

Be prepared

Gather information on the extent of the problem, with specific examples. Seek out collaborative evidence from other friends and family. Develop a list of unacceptable behaviors and consequences the person should expect if they occur. Research OUD and treatment options so you're ready with solid information.

Consider whom your loved one might listen to

Think about involving a trusted friend or relative who's also concerned. This may be a parent, sibling, close friend, grandparent or teacher. Consider having a meeting to make plans with the people you intend to include in the intervention. Talk about the best way to handle the conversation and topics to include and avoid.

If you choose to have the discussion as a family, consider including children for the purpose of speaking about their personal experiences. However, avoid exposing young children to the more challenging parts of the conversation, such as in-depth discussions on behavioral expectations and next steps.

You might also consider asking someone who's not in your family to help guide the discussion if you feel that would reduce confrontation, especially if you expect strong emotional responses.

Carefully choose the time and place to talk

Don't have the conversation when the person is under the influence of drugs or alcohol. Don't have it at the end of a long workday or after something has happened that's upsetting. Choose a time when no one else is around except those taking part in the discussion. Limit distractions.

Consider holding the intervention outside your home. An addiction specialist, such as a drug and alcohol counselor, psychologist or social worker, can help arrange the best environment. These people can also guide discussions to help keep them on topic. Involving professionals can be especially helpful when you have concerns that a loved one may react in a self-destructive or violent way.

Have a plan for what to say

Have prewritten notes on what each person will say during the intervention and try to stick to the script.

Once the conversation begins, follow the plan and be intentional about what you say.

Tell the person how much you care

Begin by explaining that you're coming from a place of love and concern. "I care about you and that's why I'm doing this. Let's work on this together." Explain why you're making this effort to talk together.

Focus your responses on your worries about what will happen if things don't change. Explain to your loved one that this is an opportunity to focus on a new future together.

Use "I" statements

Approaching the conversation from your own perspective helps you avoid sounding like you're making accusations. It also helps avoid confrontation. Instead of using statements that begin with "You" — such as "You are . . . ," "You did . . . ," or "You ruined . . ." — say things like:
- "I have noticed you're struggling."
- "I can't help but wonder about some of your decisions and behaviors. Here is what I've noticed . . ."
- "I want you to . . ." (Avoid using "You should . . ." or "You need to . . .")
- "I'm concerned you may have opioid use disorder."
- "I feel scared and worried about what may happen if we don't get the help you need."

Stay calm

This is the most important and potentially the hardest thing you need to do. As the conversation continues, be patient. Your loved one is struggling and likely feels helpless and out of control. You need to stay in control.

Carefully monitor your tone of voice. Keep it even, clear, compassionate and caring. Don't raise your voice. Don't allow the conversation to escalate into a shouting match. In the heat of the moment, people often say things they don't mean or can't take back. Don't let it get to that heated level. If things get heated, stop, agree to talk about it again later and walk away so both parties can cool off.

Stay focused

At times the conversation may veer off onto different topics. Your loved one may try to distract you and others present from the topic at hand. Be sure to bring the conversation back to the main issue.

Share facts and feelings

Talk to your loved one about the signs, behaviors and reactions you've observed that concern you. Make the experience personal. Ask each person to talk about how the addiction has affected them personally, including emotional and financial problems. Use facts as much as possible. It's hard to argue with facts.

Explain the consequences of their addiction

Ask whether your loved one has noticed these consequences. Your loved one may not recognize the negative effects their behaviors have had on themselves and others.

Don't walk on eggshells

Be honest, open and very frank. Speak the truth even if it's hard. Don't push facts or the problems under the rug.

Be prepared to be blamed

Taking responsibility for bad behavior isn't easy. Your loved one may make accusations and try to turn the focus on others. The focus is usually turned on the person raising the concern.

Stay calm and continue going back to the plan. Stick with the facts and continue to use "I" statements as much as possible.

Set safe boundaries

You and your family may be at risk. Examples of risky situations include drug dealing from the home, using injectable opioids, driving while under the influence and engaging in criminal activities. These shouldn't be tolerated and should have immediate consequences.

Use the conversation to set firm limits on activities that are completely unacceptable and lay out consequences for not complying. This can be one of the most difficult parts of the conversation.

End the conversation by proposing treatment options

Come to the conversation prepared to talk about treatment options. Do your research and be ready to share information. Refer to Chapters 12 and 13 for details about treatment and how to find a program.

Ask for an immediate decision

Your loved one may be most likely to agree to treatment if held accountable for choosing an option on the spot. He or she may ask for time to think things over, but this could increase the risk of pursuing even more dangerous behaviors or delaying a decision. If your loved one

DISCUSS NALOXONE

Friends and family taking part in an intervention are likely to be the ones who witness an overdose if it happens. Consider using this time to talk about naloxone. Chapter 6 explains how people can obtain naloxone, when to use it and who's at greatest risk. Appendix F lists the specific steps to administer naloxone along with other emergency care.

agrees to start treatment, make sure you follow through on plans quickly.

Describe how you'll help make treatment a success

This may include providing financial support, caring for young children that are involved, taking your loved one to treatment sessions and participating in therapy.

DRAWING THE LINE

Just like fences set physical boundaries for where you should and shouldn't go, healthy relationships need boundaries to keep thoughts and actions in check.

The breakdown of emotional and physical boundaries is a hallmark of addiction. Every activity linked to addiction that impacts other family members runs the risk of crossing a healthy boundary. To combat this, friends and family should draw firm boundaries defining what is and isn't acceptable.

Boundaries can be set at the time of an intervention or even earlier if necessary. It can be helpful to write a list of all the boundaries you set and the consequences for crossing them.

Here are some examples of problems that may develop and suggested boundaries for dealing with them.
- **Problem:** Shouting or uncontrolled verbal outbursts with hurtful comments.

- **Response:** "I'm setting boundaries around how you can treat me and our family. If you shout or make hurtful comments, I'll leave the room and the conversation ends. We can talk another time when you're in control of your emotions."

- **Problem:** Drug-related activities that put the family's safety at risk.
- **Response:** "I'm setting boundaries around what activities can take place in our home. Your use of drugs in the house puts everyone at risk. You won't be able to live at home if you continue to use drugs here."

- **Problem:** People coming to the home who put the family's safety at risk.
- **Response:** "I'm setting boundaries around the people coming into our house that I feel aren't a good influence on you or other members of the household. If they come to the house, they'll be asked to leave."

- **Problem:** Enabling drug-related activities.
- **Response:** "I'm setting boundaries around activities that I feel make your addiction worse. I will no longer make excuses for your behaviors." Then provide some specific examples of how you've done this, such as driving to different health care providers in an attempt to get more opioids for the person.

More on enabling

Enabling is doing things that make it easier for a loved one to continue self-destructive patterns of behavior. When it comes to opioids, it means helping people avoid facing the negative consequences of their addiction.

Examples of enabling include:
- Taking your loved one to appointments with multiple doctors (doctor shopping) to obtain pain medications.
- Being dishonest with health care providers about use of opioids at home.
- Compensating for the roles your loved one no longer fulfills.
- Making excuses for absences at school, work and family gatherings.
- Not following through on the consequences that you have set for dangerous behaviors.

Most often, you're trying to protect the person and keep things working in the family and in your relationship. This is

---

SAFETY IS A PRIORITY

Sometimes, someone who struggles with addiction lives a lifestyle that causes unsafe living conditions for you and others. Your safety and the safety of those in your household takes priority over all other issues.

Consider other living arrangements if activities related to OUD are putting anyone in your home at risk.

natural. But when someone struggles with addiction, enabling isn't helpful.

There's only so much that you can do to protect people from their own actions. Many times, people who use opioids continue to do so despite understanding they're breaking household rules, engaging in criminal activities or placing their own health at risk.

This part will likely be the hardest thing you do. You may need to allow bad things to happen so your loved one experiences the consequences of their actions and bad choices. Your inclination may be to step in and save the day. But what you're really doing is helping your loved one avoid facing the negative consequences of addiction.

When rules are broken, try to follow through on the consequences you've set. This may help your loved one realize the extreme nature of their circumstances. At that point, they may be willing to consider treatment.

If you're not sure whether your actions are helpful, talk to your own health care provider, trusted loved ones or support groups.

LET'S PRACTICE

It may be difficult to picture yourself having this type of conversation. Most people avoid confrontation, so tackling a topic as charged as substance abuse is likely to bring out a lot of strong emotions. Keep in mind the reasons you're having the intervention — to save a life and preserve a relationship.

Sometimes rehearsing the intervention in your mind can be a helpful way to prepare for the real event.

To give you an idea of how an intervention might look, here is an example scenario.

The situation

John is 54 years old and has a history of chronic low back pain following a car accident six months ago. His primary care provider initially prescribed oxycodone for two weeks to help manage severe pain after the injury. After the first prescription ran out, the provider recommended physical therapy and a combination of acetaminophen and ibuprofen.

John didn't want to try these treatments and began to seek opioid prescriptions from other providers. He went to three emergency rooms requesting pain medications.

John's wife, Susan, noticed he was taking opioids daily and more frequently than what was indicated on the prescription labels. He stopped taking part in activities he enjoyed, such as golfing and fishing.

John also spent more time sleeping. Susan was concerned about the time he spent trying to get opioids. She worried about the side effects of the drugs. He was late to work many times because he overslept.

Susan suggested to John that he consider cutting back on the opioids. He became angry and stormed out of the house.

Friends and family told Susan, "John just isn't himself these days."

Susan believes John has developed an addiction to opioids. After consulting her own health care provider, family members and a social worker, she's decided to do an intervention. She has researched opioids and treatment programs. She bought a notebook and wrote notes about what she wants to discuss. She made plans with family. Everyone knows what each of them will say.

Take a look inside John and Susan's home and listen to this intervention.

Location: The family living room

Who is in the room: John; Susan; John's parents, Rich and Lynn; and John and Susan's 16-year-old daughter, Robyn

The conversation

Susan, in a calm, controlled and concerned tone:
John, we're all here because we love you and we're concerned about you. As a family, we would like to discuss your opioid use.

John:
What about it?

Susan:
We've noticed you're taking opioids differently from how they were prescribed. I feel you're just not yourself when you take them. I've also noticed that you aren't doing the things you normally like to do. You've told me your pain isn't better when you take

opioids. *You don't seem to be able to do any new things you couldn't do without the opioids. We're all truly concerned you've become addicted to them.*

John, sounding defensive and angry:
Addicted! We've been married 22 years. You know me better than anyone else. How could you even say something like this? This conversation is utterly ridiculous, and I'm done with it.

Susan, in a calm voice:
John, please know I'm not bringing this up because I'm angry. I'm genuinely scared for your health. I feel you've become less reliable when I need you. And I feel like the drugs are the most important thing to you right now, more important than me, our marriage and our daughter.

John, getting angrier and louder:
Listen, you know I struggle with pain. I'm the victim in all of this. Do you think I want to live the way I do? You're just like the rest of these so-called health care people. You think you know how to solve my problems when the truth is you don't understand them at all. I thought you were on my side! I thought all of you were on my side!

Susan, staying calm and patient:
John, I'm on your side, which is why I feel so strongly about talking about this. We're all on your side and that's why we're here.

John:
Well, you sure don't act like it. It's like you want me to be in pain. You take away my meds and then what? Do you plan on letting me suffer? Those pills are the only thing keeping me going right now.

Susan:

I know this conversation isn't easy, but I think it's important that you hear everyone's perspective on this. I'll let the others here share their thoughts with you.

Lynn:

John, you know how much I love you. You used to call me twice a week, but the past three months, I've only heard from you twice. I miss you, son. I worry those opioids are taking my son from me.

Robyn:

I'm worried about you too, Dad. We used to spend time together. You always seem busy now or like you don't feel good. You don't help me with my homework anymore. You even missed my science fair last week and my choir concert a few weeks ago. You make excuses and you make promises you don't keep.

Susan:

Honey, I don't see you living. I don't see you active or involved. Don't you want to get back to the things you loved to do, to the people you loved doing them with? Is this the life you want to keep living?

John, begrudgingly:

Well, maybe I could cut back on the pills some.

Susan:

John, I spoke about my concerns with your doctor. You know he's talked with you about not taking opioids for your back. He suggested other ways to help with your pain, but you weren't willing to even give them a try. You seem to be more interested in getting the opioids than making your pain

better. The doctor would like to meet with you this week to talk about a condition called opioid use disorder. He knows how to treat it.

John, shocked and angry:

You don't have any right to talk to my doctor!

Susan, staying calm:

Your doctor is as worried about you as we are. I don't want you to be a statistic, John. I've read a lot about opioid use disorder and the statistics are scary. When you get so sleepy, I am scared that one day, you just won't wake up.

I'm not going to keep helping you put yourself and our family at risk. I'm setting some boundaries. I'm not driving you to emergency rooms anymore or filling more opioid prescriptions. I am no longer OK with you passing out on the couch during the day in front of our daughter. And I don't want you driving when you take opioids. You could hurt yourself or someone else.

John:

So, what is it that you want me to do?

Susan:

First, I want to start by both of us meeting with your doctor. Your doctor already gave me a list of treatment programs for OUD. I've done some homework and found two within a 15-minute drive. I've called the insurance company to make sure the programs are in-network.

John, know that we're all going to help you through this every step of the way. You don't have to do this by yourself. But we need to *know today that you will commit to this plan, a plan to get better.*

John:
I suppose you're not giving me much choice.

Susan:
But it's the right choice. We love you, John. We know this isn't easy, but we'll get through this together. We are partners in this. You won't be going through this alone.

Reflections

Notice how in this dialogue, Susan stayed calm, organized and patient. She stuck to her plan. She used "I" statements. She set boundaries. She kept her part of the conversation genuine, calm and compassionate.

Susan had done her research and was ready to respond when John seemed willing to get help for OUD. She did not let John's defensiveness and anger distract from the goal of the intervention. She kept reminding him all this effort was because she loved him.

Sadly, most interventions don't go this smoothly. Remember, these can be very confrontational situations. If the first time doesn't go as planned, don't give up!

If you've held an intervention that didn't work, mentally replay the scenario and see where things seemed to fall apart.
• Did you go off the topic?
• Did you feel blamed and then give in to the pressure to end the discussion too soon?

• Did you come with enough facts to make your case?
• Were the right people present? If not, who could help the next time you try?

Knowing where the discussion got derailed can prepare you for the next one. Treatment is a journey, not a destination. Keep yourself and your loved ones safe — and try again another time.

Helping a loved one make important changes can be very difficult. Consider talking to your own health care provider for advice. Partner with someone who can share important information about addiction, prescribe medications and make referrals to outside treatments as needed.

When everyone works together, this leads to the greatest chance of recovery.

———————— **W H A T I F** ————————

sharing your truth becomes their path to freedom?

14

What if . . . ?

The opioid epidemic is a story about all of us. It's about the people we love, the people we've lost and the people we fear losing. Whether the stories we have shared come from friends, family or total strangers, they're all passed on with a purpose: to educate and plead for change, to pave the path for a different tomorrow.

The stories beg us to ask this question: What if . . . ?

It's a powerful inquiry. We can use this simple question to reflect on the past, present and future all at once. For many of you reading this book, finding the answer to a "what-if" question is the very reason you picked up the book.

- "What if my pain gets so bad, I choose to take two tramadol pills instead of one? Could something bad happen?"

- "What if I choose to use opioids for more than a month? Does my risk of addiction increase?"
- "What if I decided to confront my wife about how many oxycodone pills she takes? Will this destroy our relationship?"
- "What if I'd just thrown away my leftover opioids instead of leaving them unlocked in my medicine cabinet? Would my grandchild still be alive?"
- "What if I took a more active role in a pain management plan? Could I avoid complications from opioids?"

If you've pondered these kinds of questions more than once, you're not alone. The world of opioids can be confusing and contradictory. Our nation has grappled with balancing the medicinal powers of opioids with their toxic enticements. We've watched the pendulum swing to and fro as we've liberalized their use to manage pain, and then reined them back in to deal with their destructive side effects.

What if we're the last generation to battle the drugs for control? What if we choose to solve our current problems?

This is your opportunity.

The purpose of this book is to empower you to answer your "what-ifs" and use that information to make safe, informed decisions. Below we offer a summary of the most common "what-if" situations you may find yourself in. We hope this book offers you guidance on next steps to take to find freedom, hope and healing.

If these situations don't apply to you, consider passing on the knowledge you've gained as a resource to friends, family and colleagues. When we are well equipped and well informed, we can change the world.

WHAT IF YOU'RE IN PAIN AND BEING PRESCRIBED OPIOIDS?

Chapters 4 through 8 give you an overview of pain and how to use opioids safely to manage your pain. No matter the type or source of pain you have, here are a few key steps to follow to help keep you safe:

- **Include others.** When you talk with your health care provider, you may have a hard time remembering all the details of your visit, especially if you're in pain. Bring a trusted friend or family member to the discussion to help fill in your story, remember treatment plans and advocate for you if needed.

- **Talk about alternatives.** Don't be afraid to ask questions about whether you really need opioids. As you've read, taking opioids should also be paired with nonopioid treatments. If they aren't being offered, ask why.
- **Understand the goal.** The goal of treatment with opioids is to function better, not completely take away your pain. Ask your health care provider these questions:
  - Do I really need opioids?
  - What are other options to manage pain instead of opioids?
  - What are the side effects of the opioids I'm being prescribed?
  - Do I have risk factors that put me at greater risk of side effects?
  - Exactly when and how should I take the opioid?
  - What are my goals with this treatment?
  - What are the next steps if the pain is not getting better despite the treatment?
  - Do I need to have my drugs tapered when I stop taking them?
  - Do I need to keep naloxone on hand?
  - What is the first thing I should do if I have concerns about becoming addicted to opioids?

- **Use exactly as prescribed.** Always take the medications exactly as prescribed. Remember, you don't have to finish the bottle of opioids if pain is getting better.
- **Don't "doctor shop."** Ideally, only one health care provider should prescribe opioids for you. This is the safest way to ensure you take only exactly what you need and avoid dangerous drug interactions.

- **Don't share.** Never share your prescriptions with other people or take other people's medications.
- **Store opioids safely.** Always store opioids and other medications (including your children's) away from where people can access them, preferably in a locked location.
- **Dispose of opioids safely.** Don't save your remaining opioids for another time you might have pain. Once you're done taking them, follow the instructions in this book for safely disposing of them.
- **Keep naloxone on hand.** If you're at risk of an opioid-related overdose, your provider may prescribe naloxone. Keep it with you at all times. So that others are aware that you take opioids, consider wearing a medical alert bracelet. The bracelet helps others know you are at risk for opioid-related complications.
- **Build a good relationship with your provider.** Some health care providers may ask questions about your past use of opioids or review your risk factors. This may be an uncomfortable conversation. Your provider may also require screening tests, such as urine drug screens or pill counts. Remember, these steps are taken for your safety.
- **Know the signs of OUD.** Watch for them when using opioids and act quickly.
- **Speak up.** If you're concerned that your health care provider isn't prescribing opioids safely, mention it to them. Remember, one treatment plan doesn't work for everyone. If you continue to have concerns, get another opinion or find another provider.
- **Encourage opioid stewardship.** Opioid stewardship programs (OSP) can be an effective way for health care institutions to promote best practices when it comes to opioids. Ask your health care provider if their practice has an established OSP and encourage development if one doesn't exist. Read Appendix A to learn more about opioid stewardship programs.

WHAT IF YOU'RE WORRIED YOU HAVE OUD?

If you're worried that you may have an addiction to opioids, follow these steps:
- **Tell your loved ones.** Telling trusted loved ones about your concerns is the first step. Your loved ones may already have the same concerns and may be able to help with next steps.
- **Tell your health care provider.** Your provider can do screening tests, arrange treatment referrals and prescribe medications to control the disorder.
- **Get treatment.** Partner with your health care team, other community resources or loved ones to support you while you get the help you need.
- **Ask about MOUD.** When you explore treatments, ask whether MOUD is included in the treatment plan.
- **Seek treatment for all parts of the disorder.** Ask your treatment team about the types of therapies included in your treatment plan and whether they include a biopsychosocial approach.

WHAT IF YOU'RE IN RECOVERY FROM OUD?

Recovery takes time and there often are hurdles and setbacks along the way.

- **If you fall, get back up.** As you read earlier, relapse is common, especially if treatment is too short or fails to address other causes related to your disorder. Remember, relapse is the norm, not the exception — so don't give up! Have a relapse-prevention plan in place for when this happens, including knowing whom to call and what to do next.
- **Rebuild relationships.** Friends and family may have been hurt by things you've said or done when struggling with addiction. Make rebuilding healthy relationships a priority.
- **Rejoin life.** Because OUD can destroy so many parts of your life such as jobs, finances and relationships, it's easy to become isolated. The point of recovery is to get your life back. Don't be afraid to take back what the disorder has taken from you. Find a supportive work environment, work with financial advisers and engage in safe activities that bring joy and rebuild relationships.
- **Join a support network.** There are many support programs for people recovering from OUD, such as Narcotics Anonymous, Celebrate Recovery and others offered through treatment programs, the community and faith communities. Staying engaged with others in recovery helps prevent relapse and promote healthy relationships.
- **Share your success.** Your recovery story is powerful. It may be the motivation someone else needs to begin their own recovery journey. Consider seeking opportunities to help others struggling with their addiction, such as through community and state-sponsored events or those hosted through treatment programs.

I know there are no simple answers to the complex questions about opioids. Hopefully, we can find a way to make a difference. It's got to be a team effort between a lot of different people. We simply have to do better.

PATRICK D. MCGOWAN, MINNEAPOLIS POLICE DEPARTMENT (RET.), MINNESOTA STATE SENATOR (RET.) AND HENNEPIN COUNTY SHERIFF (RET.)

- **Be an advocate.** Talk to community leaders, law enforcement officials and lawmakers about your personal opioid journey. Share your insight, offer solutions and ask how you can get engaged to help support prevention and recovery efforts.

WHAT IF A LOVED ONE IS USING OR MISUSING OPIOIDS?

One of the most powerful tools we have against the opioid epidemic is each other. You can make a difference and save a life. If a loved one is currently taking opioids or struggling with opioid-related complications:
- **Know the signs of OUD.** Talk to your loved one's health care provider right away if you believe your loved one has OUD.

- **Set safe and healthy boundaries.** If OUD is affecting relationships or the safety of people in your home, set firm boundaries to keep everyone safe.
- **Encourage treatment.** Work with your loved one to find an appropriate treatment program that works. Make phone calls, do the research and help deal with insurance issues.
- **Stay engaged.** Ask to go with your loved one to provider appointments. Take notes, ask questions, understand risks and benefits and make sure your loved one understands them as well.
- **Provide emotional support.** People often voice frustrations, share concerns and look for empathy from loved ones. Offer a supportive, listening ear. You can help your loved one focus on the big picture and offer a hopeful outlook that keeps him or her motivated to pursue helpful treatments.
- **Be an advocate.** People do not always speak up for themselves. Be your loved one's voice when you see safety concerns or unmet needs.
- **Know the signs of an overdose and be prepared to act.** Make sure that you have naloxone on hand and know how to give it if needed.
- **Keep the care team together.** It's easy to become overwhelmed when seeking treatment. Help your loved one stay in contact with his or her primary care provider while receiving treatment from other medical providers.
- **Support recovery from relapses.** If your loved one relapses, don't turn away. Offer reassuring and encouraging support while still maintaining firm boundaries.

MARY: "SHE WOULD STILL BE HERE"

I ask myself, "What if . . . ?" all the time.

What if I had questioned my mom's continued use of opioids? What if I had encouraged her to find another way to help with the knee pain? What if I had gone with her to doctor's appointments so I could speak up and advocate for something besides opioids?

I know the answer: She would still be here.

She would have seen her granddaughter play the lead in her high school musical. She would have seen her graduate from high school. She would have seen my brother succeed in his career and know he is happy now and doing well. She would have gone with me to quilt shows. She would have sat on my front porch in the white rocker and visited with me while I planted spring flowers. She would have known her great-grandson.

"What if . . ." doesn't do any good when it's too late. I do know I can't go back and change things. But I can try to make things different for others.

So can you.

- **Join support groups.** Ask about available support groups for family members of people with OUD. Consider attending a support group if you're able.

WHAT IF WE ALL WORKED TOGETHER?

If the end of this book marks the beginning of a new chapter in your life, then the book will have accomplished its goals. People are powerful when informed. It's time to be an ambassador. Take this opportunity to share the knowledge you've learned with those who need it most. Partnership is the foundation for solving the problems caused by this epidemic.

Medical providers can't prescribe us out of the opioid crisis. Government agencies can't regulate us out of it. Drug treatment programs can't counsel us out of it. This book can impart knowledge, yet knowledge without action won't end this crisis either. We all need to do our part. We must all work together.

Hope is in sight and the crisis is ours to end. The ending must include you.

——————— **W H A T   I F** ———————

*we are the generation
that ends this epidemic
for good?*

Additional resources

Mayo Clinic Pain Rehabilitation Center
www.mayoclinic.org/departments-centers/
pain-rehabilitation-center

American Chronic Pain Association
www.theacpa.org

Substance Abuse and Mental Health Services Administration (SAMHSA): Behavioral Health Treatment Services Locator
www.findtreatment.samhsa.gov

National Helpline
1-800-662-HELP (4357)

Health and Human Services (HHS): Find Opioid Treatment Programs
www.hhs.gov/opioids/treatment/index.html

Mayo Clinic Addiction Services, Rochester, Minnesota
www.mayoclinic.org/departments-centers/
psychiatry/addiction-services/overview

U.S. Food and Drug Administration (FDA): Where and how to dispose of unused medicines
www.fda.gov/consumers/consumer-updates/
where-and-how-dispose-unused-medicines

DEA Diversion Control Division: Drug Disposal Information
www.deadiversion.usdoj.gov/
drug_disposal/index.html

Centers for Disease Control and Prevention (CDC): Opioids
www.cdc.gov/opioids/index.html

National Suicide Prevention Lifeline
Call 988 or 800-273-8255

Crisis Text Line
Text HOME to 741741

About Mayo Clinic efforts to address the opioid crisis

In 2016, drug overdoses took more American lives than the number of lives lost during the Vietnam and Iraq wars combined. With opioids contributing to an estimated 60% or more of all drug overdoses, it was clear that we were losing the deadliest drug battle in American history. The most severe opioid-related complications — addiction and overdose deaths — were impacting our family members, our neighbors, our friends and our colleagues.

Recognizing the critical importance of mounting an aggressive, proactive response, in 2017, Mayo Clinic mobilized one of the largest enterprise task forces in its history to objectively appraise and address the crisis.

The group's responsibilities included addressing best practices for pain management; performing quality analytics on internal opioid prescribing behaviors; developing protocols, procedures and workflows for safe opioid prescribing; building both patient and provider educational tools; and ensuring proper prevention and management of opioid-related complications.

Over a span of four years, the steward-ship group made substantial efforts to study internal prescribing behaviors, opioid consumption patterns of Mayo Clinic patients and complication rates of various regimens. The group surveyed Mayo Clinic staff, patients and community members. Stewardship group members reviewed high-quality literature and solicited opinions from experts around the country. Every opinion mattered.

As a result of this assessment, health care personnel participated in required education on effective prescribing practices. Robust internal policies and workflows offered safety nets to support adherence and appropriate referrals. Videos, educational resources and electronic diaries were developed for patients so they could make informed decisions. Resources about opioids and pain management weren't just revised; they were completely scrapped and written anew to reflect important messages.

Mayo Clinic's commitment to change didn't end at our organization's borders. Group leaders were given the important responsibility of presenting the program's components to state and federal partners, national task forces and regulatory bodies involved in addressing the opioid epidemic. The stewardship group shared collective knowledge with the broader medical community through national presentations, videos and podcasts.

Emerging from this response was the award-winning Opioid Stewardship Program, which has achieved national attention for its comprehensive, patient-centered infrastructure.

To date, this stewardship program remains one of the largest and most well-established opioid stewardship programs in the country. The team is dedicated to ensuring that Mayo Clinic prescribes opioids to the right person, for the right reason, in the right form, at the right dose and for the right length of treatment.

The program's goal is to educate the people most likely to turn the tide of this epidemic. We believe this includes you. This book represents one of our many efforts to provide our patients and communities with the tools they need to be informed. Through partnership and collaboration, we can be the last generation to fight this battle.

For more information about how to establish a robust stewardship program, review the information found on the website for the American Hospital Association called Stem the Tide: Addressing the Opioid Epidemic and Taking Action. Here is the URL: www.aha.org/guidesreports/ 2017-11-07-stem-tide-addressing-opioid-epidemic-taking-action

What is pharmacogenomics?

Pharmacogenomics (PGx) is the study of how your genes may affect the way your body responds to, or interacts with, some medications.

Genes are inherited from your biological parents. They carry information that determines characteristics such as eye color and blood type. Genes can also influence how you process and respond to medications.

PGx testing is one tool your health care team can use to help identify the right medication for you.

WHAT FACTORS AFFECT YOUR RESPONSE TO MEDICATIONS?

Several factors affect how a person responds to medications, including:
- Genetic factors.
- Age.
- Sex.
- Race/ethnicity.
- Illness or problems with organ function, especially kidney or liver function.
- Smoking and alcohol use.
- Food interactions.
- Other medications.

WHY MIGHT PGX TESTING BE RECOMMENDED OR CONSIDERED?

A health care provider may order PGx

testing to help guide your current or future medication use, such as:

- To avoid or prevent serious side effects related to certain medications.
- To adjust the dose of a current medication or recommend a different medication.
- To identify a medication or dose of a medication most likely to work for you.

HOW ARE PGX RESULTS USED?

A health care provider may recommend you have PGx testing and use the results to help create a pain treatment plan. Because medications are processed differently by the body, gene testing helps health care providers select medications most

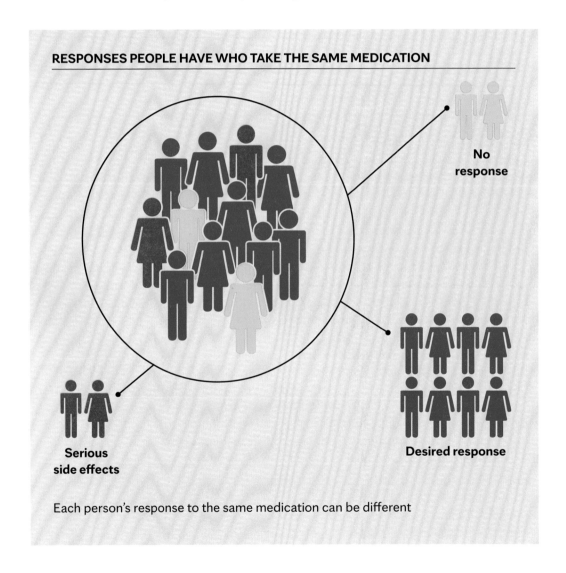

RESPONSES PEOPLE HAVE WHO TAKE THE SAME MEDICATION

No response

Serious side effects

Desired response

Each person's response to the same medication can be different likely to provide pain relief with the fewest side effects.

HOW IS PGX TESTING DONE?

To get a sample for PGx testing, a health care provider collects one of the following:
- A small sample of blood.
- A small sample of saliva.
- A cheek swab.

IS PGX TESTING COVERED BY INSURANCE?

Some insurance companies may cover PGx testing, depending on their policies and the reasons for testing. Contact your insurance provider about coverage before you're tested if this is a concern.

CAN PGX TESTING RESULTS AFFECT INSURANCE COVERAGE?

The Genetic Information Nondiscrimination Act prohibits medical insurance companies and employers from discriminating against people on the basis of genetic information. This includes PGx test results.

To learn more about the Genetic Information Nondiscrimination Act, go to this URL: www.genome.gov/about-genomics/policy-issues/Genetic-Discrimination

ABOUT PGX TESTING RESULTS

When you receive your results:
- Don't make any changes to the medications or the dosages of medications you take without talking to your health care provider or pharmacist.
- Share your results with all your health care providers as part of your personal health history.
- Be aware that PGx results provide guidelines for some medications.
- Know that PGx testing doesn't:
  - Apply to all medications.
  - Address all medication side effects or medication allergies.
  - Explain drug-drug interactions or drug-food interactions.

PGx results are specific to only the person being tested. Don't use your PGx results to guide medication decisions for others, even family members.

Questions to ask when considering a treatment program

Bring this book with you when you meet to discuss treatment programs. Use it to ensure that you ask the questions to get the answers you need. Record the answers.

Sometimes, the amount of information you're given can be overwhelming. Consider bringing someone with you when you meet with program staff so you both can hear the responses and talk about it later.

Important questions to ask include:

☐ Does the program offer a spectrum of treatment environments? If yes, what criteria are used to move people between treatment environments?

☐ Does the program offer a spectrum of treatment services? If yes, which treatments are available through the program?

☐ What types of services would need to be sought outside the program?

☐ Are all the providers who offer services in your program licensed?

☐ What does the program cost?

☐ Can I get an estimate of daily, weekly and monthly service costs?

- [ ] What treatments are included in these costs?

- [ ] Are there other costs related to mental health services, medical care and room and board for inpatient environments?

- [ ] Are there additional fees for detox or aftercare?

- [ ] Is the program covered by insurance?

- [ ] When I call the insurance company, are there specific terms I should use to ask about coverage?

- [ ] How does the program track its success rates?

- [ ] What are the rates for each of these?
  - [ ] Program dropout.
  - [ ] Recovery.
  - [ ] Relapse.
  - [ ] Employment.
  - [ ] Criminal activity.
  - [ ] Overdose.
  - [ ] Client satisfaction.

- [ ] What goals does the program use to assess and track progress?

- [ ] How does the program set and monitor participants' goals within the program?

- [ ] How can family members or friends collaborate with program staff to support these goals?

- [ ] What are the program's relapse policies?

- [ ] What are the policies regarding communication with friends and families while in treatment? At what point during treatment do these rules change?

- [ ] Does the program arrange community transition and aftercare?

- [ ] Who prescribes MOUD once someone is discharged from the program?

Glossary

abstinence. Abstinence means to not do something, to abstain. In relation to opioids, it means to not use opioids at all.

addiction. Addiction is a chronic condition that impacts medical, psychological, social and spiritual functions to the point that people have difficulty managing their lives and controlling their behaviors.

aftercare treatment program. Aftercare treatment is follow-up support and treatment after the completion of an addiction treatment program.

allodynia. Allodynia occurs when nerve impulses from nonpainful stimuli, such as a light touch, are perceived as pain.

amygdala. The amygdala is the part of the brain that contributes to feelings of stress, unease, anxiety and agitation. It's a brain area designed to let other areas of your brain know that things aren't well with you.

antagonist. Antagonists are medications that completely block cell receptors without activating them. Opioid antagonists block opioid cell receptors. An example of an antagonist is naltrexone.

antidepressants. Antidepressants are a class of medication that affects the processing and signaling of neurotransmitters that regulate both mood and pain sensations. They're particularly helpful for chronic pain conditions, such as fibromyalgia and migraine headaches. Examples include tricyclic antidepressants, selective serotonin reuptake inhibitors and serotonin-norepinephrine reuptake inhibitors.

benzodiazepines. Benzodiazepines are a class of medications prescribed to treat anxiety, insomnia and seizures. Taking benzodiazepines with opioids increases the risk of overdose due to the potential of both medications to cause sleepiness and difficulty breathing. Examples include diazepam (Valium), lorazepam (Ativan), clonazepam (Klonopin) and alprazolam (Xanax).

Centers for Disease Control and Prevention. The CDC is a federal public health agency in the U.S. Department of Health and Human Services that detects and responds to new and emerging health threats, advances science and technology to prevent disease, and promotes healthy and safe behaviors, among other responsibilities.

central sensitization. Central sensitization is a condition in which someone experiences increased sensitivity and over-responsiveness of the central nervous system to sensory stimulation, including pain.

compulsion. Compulsion is the irresistible urge to behave in a certain manner, even against a person's own wishes and values.

controlled substance. Controlled substances are federally regulated and can only be prescribed or administered by people with a license to do so. Opioids are a controlled substance.

COX-2 inhibitors. COX-2 inhibitors are a class of medication that selectively inhibits the COX-2 enzyme, reducing overall inflammation. The only currently available COX-2 inhibitor in the U.S. is celecoxib (Celebrex).

dependence. Dependence refers to physical or psychological symptoms that make people feel like they must continue to take a substance.

detoxification (detox). Detox is the process of eliminating addictive substances from the body and managing withdrawal symptoms.

Diagnostic and Statistical Manual of Mental Disorders (DSM-5). The DSM-5 lists criteria that providers can use to diagnose opioid use disorder.

doctor shopping. Doctor shopping is the practice of seeing multiple doctors in an effort to receive a desired service or medication.

dopamine. Dopamine is the pleasure chemical released by the brain. Opioids increase dopamine release to much higher levels than the brain typically releases with everyday pleasurable activities, such as socializing with friends and eating ice cream.

drug courts. Drug courts refer to legal court processes established for people with substance use disorder. Drug courts often offer substance abuse treatment in place of jail sentences.

drug diversion. Drug diversion occurs when someone uses a controlled substance that's prescribed for someone else.

drug elimination. Drug elimination is the process of a drug being removed from the body through the body's normal waste system. This is sometimes referred to as clearing the drug from the body.

drug inactivation. Inactivation is the process of turning a drug into a form that the body doesn't use.

enabling. Enabling behaviors make it easier for a loved one to continue self-destructive patterns of behavior. With opioids, it means helping someone access drugs or avoid facing the negative consequences of their addiction.

epidemic. An epidemic is a problem with sudden rapid spread and growth affecting many people.

epigenetics. This term describes the process of environmental factors inducing long-term changes in how a gene ultimately functions. Environmental factors include living circumstances, traumatic experiences, drug access and stress. This phenomenon can greatly affect how someone responds and adapts to opioid use.

euphoria. Euphoria is the feeling or state of intense excitement and happiness, often described as feeling high or getting a rush. People who experience euphoria with opioids are more likely to develop addiction with recurrent use.

extended-release (ER) medications. ER medications are designed to release slowly into the bloodstream at a steady concentration over long periods of time. They're also called sustained-release (SR) medications.

fentanyl test strips. These small strips of paper are capable of detecting fentanyl contamination in drugs.

gabapentinoids. This class of medication works primarily by reducing inappropriate nerve conduction. Examples include gabapentin and pregabalin.

harm reduction. Harm reduction is an evidence-based strategy with the goal of reducing death, injury, disease, overdose and substance use disorder. The strategy includes making syringe service programs, fentanyl test strips and naloxone readily available.

hyperalgesia. Hyperalgesia occurs when the body begins to perceive pain in an overly exaggerated manner. Things that usually hurt just a little hurt much more.

illicit drugs. Illicit drugs are those obtained without a prescription or for no legitimate medical reason. They're also called illegal drugs or street drugs.

immediate-release (IR) medications. IR medications are absorbed into the body quickly.

immunosuppression. Immunosuppression is the partial or complete suppression of the immune response of a person's body. It may be caused by disease and medications.

in-network providers. These are health care providers that insurance companies have contracted with to provide services for certain fees. Services from in-network providers are more likely to be covered by insurance.

inpatient treatment programs. These programs provide short- or long-term living environments. They're also called residential treatment programs.

integrative therapies. Integrative therapies are mind-body treatments that may be used to manage pain. Integrative therapies target the biopsychosocial roots of the pain, addressing the whole person, including mind, body and spirit.

intervention. An intervention is a planned conversation focused on getting a person to seek treatment for addiction. An intervention can be done by family, friends, health care providers or addiction specialists.

medical coping. Medical coping is use of a drug to reduce or relieve psychological pain.

medications for opioid use disorder (**MOUD**). MOUD is a biologic treatment approach using specific opioids to treat opioid use disorder. It's also called medication assisted treatment (MAT). Opioids used in MOUD include methadone, buprenorphine and naltrexone.

mesolimbic pathway. The mesolimbic pathway is the part of the brain that connects brain areas closely linked with the motivation to experience pleasure. This pathway is also known as the reward circuit.

naloxone. This medication rapidly — but temporarily — reverses an opioid overdose.

nerve recruitment. In this process within the central nervous system, sensory nerves recruit nearby nerves to help process sensory information, such as touch, movement, temperature and sound. This process contributes to central sensitization.

neuroplasticity. This is the ability of nerve networks in the brain to adapt.

nonsteroid anti-inflammatory drugs (**NSAIDs**). This class of medication reduces fever, inflammation and pain. NSAIDs regulate inflammatory proteins in the blood, as well as some aspects of blood clotting. Examples include aspirin, naproxen, ibuprofen, diclofenac and ketorolac.

opiates. Opiates are naturally occurring drugs that come from the opium poppy plant, such as morphine, codeine and the illegal drug heroin.

opioid receptor. Opioid receptors are located in the outer membrane of nerve cells. Opioid medications attach to the receptors, allowing the effects of the drugs to occur, including releasing neurotransmitters such as dopamine.

opioid stewardship. This is the process of committing to safe opioid prescribing, improved outcomes and reduced misuse of opioids.

opioids. Opioids are a powerful class of medications meant to be used only for a short time to manage acute pain and improve activity levels. Opioids include both naturally occurring and lab-created opioids, also known as synthetic or semi-synthetic opioids. Examples include morphine, oxycodone, hydrocodone, hydromorphone, fentanyl and the illegal drug heroin.

opioid treatment agreement (OTA). An OTA is a document signed by patients and health care providers to work together toward a safe and effective pain management plan.

opioid use, acute. Acute opioid use is short-term use of opioids, typically for hours or days.

opioid use, chronic. Chronic use is long-term use of opioids, such as more than 45 to 90 days and on a near-daily basis.

opioid use disorder (OUD). Often shortened to "OUD," this is the name for the condition in which a person is addicted to opioids.

oral morphine equivalent (OME). This formula simplifies the dosage conversion process when a person switches from one opioid to another. Providers use a value on a chart to perform the conversion, called a morphine milligram equivalent.

orbitofrontal cortex. The orbitofrontal cortex is the part of the brain that communicates with other parts of the brain to identify salience, or levels of importance. With recurrent opioid use, this area of the brain begins to prioritize opioids over other things, such as family and friends.

outpatient treatment programs. These programs allow people to live at home and continue with work or school.

overdose. This means to take more than the recommended amount of a drug, which can result in breathing problems and even death.

pain, acute. Acute pain is sudden pain related to a specific cause, such as an injury, that usually gets better within days or weeks.

pain catastrophizing. To catastrophize about pain means to have exaggerated negative thoughts about it.

pain, chronic. Chronic pain is pain that lasts more than six months.

pain scale. Pain scales are communication tools used to assess the amount of pain a person is experiencing.

patient screening. Screening is an assessment to identify the potential risks of disease or treatment.

placebo. A placebo is a pill or medication that contains no medically active ingredient. It's often given during research studies so subjects don't know whether they're receiving the drug under study. A placebo may be given for psychological benefit if the person receiving it is likely to believe it will help.

polysubstance abuse. This occurs when people are addicted to more than one drug or substance. The use of multiple drugs or substances increases the chances of relapse after treatment.

potency. Potency is the concentration or amount of the drug needed to achieve the desired effect.

prefrontal cortex. The prefrontal cortex is the region of the brain dedicated to planning, problem-solving, decision-making and self-control. With repeated exposure to opioids, its ability to regulate other parts of the brain is diminished, leading to compulsive use of a substance with little thought to its consequences.

prescriber. Prescribers are medical professionals licensed to order (prescribe) medications and medical treatments. With reference to opioids, prescribers are health care professionals licensed to prescribe opioids and treatment for opioid addiction.

prescription drug monitoring programs (PDMPs). PDMPs are online state-run database systems that contain listings of controlled substance prescriptions filled by people in that state.

recidivism. This is the tendency of a convicted criminal to commit crimes again.

relapse. To relapse means to return to using substances after a period of sobriety.

route. Route is the manner in which a drug enters the body. Examples include swallowing, injecting and snorting. The effects of opioids are different depending on their route.

serotonin. Serotonin is a chemical released in the brain. Serotonin pathways affect mood, sleep, memory processing and cognition. Chronic opioid use distorts serotonin pathways, producing a constant state of discomfort and uneasiness.

side effect. Side effects are the secondary, usually undesirable effects of a drug or medical treatment.

sobriety. Sobriety is the state of not using substances such as opioids and alcohol.

steroids. Steroids are a class of medications that can suppress the body's immune response to injury or illness. Examples include dexamethasone, prednisone or prednisolone.

synthetic opioids. Synthetic opioids are drugs that aren't produced from naturally occurring opium poppy plants. They may be manufactured by a pharmaceutical company in a licensed laboratory or made illegally in an uncontrolled, nonmedical environment. Examples of synthetic opioids include fentanyl and methadone.

syringe service programs (SSPs). SSPs are government or privately run services that allow people using intravenous (IV) drugs to exchange used needles and syringes for new ones.

tapering. To taper off a drug means to gradually decrease the dosage. Tapering helps to prevent withdrawal symptoms, which may occur if a person stops taking a drug abruptly.

tolerance. Tolerance is the body's adjustment to a medication, requiring greater doses over time to achieve similar results.

withdrawal. Withdrawal refers to negative physical and psychological symptoms that can develop when a drug is no longer in a person's system.

Navigating insurance coverage for treatment of opioid use disorder

Health care insurance isn't always easy to figure out. The language may not be clear, and you may feel a bit lost in conversations regarding your coverage. Despite these challenges, it's important to thoroughly understand whether the cost of treatment will be covered by your insurance to avoid financial hardship and misunderstandings regarding your care.

The following information is meant to help you navigate insurance issues. If you have questions or need help, talk to a social worker from your medical facility or with a community advocacy group.

INSURANCE GLOSSARY

Here are some of the insurance terms you may encounter.

copay. A copay is the fixed amount you pay for a covered health care service after you pay your deductible. Sometimes, copays are a percentage, such as 20%, and sometimes, they're a flat fee, such as $20.

deductible. A deductible is the amount you pay for covered health care services before your insurance plan starts to pay anything. For example, if you have a $2,000 deductible, you have to pay the first $2,000 before your insurance starts to pay for submitted expenses.

explanation of benefits (EOB). An EOB is a document sent to you from your insurance company that explains how a service was covered. It includes information about the charges for a service or medication, what the insurance company paid and what you owe.

formulary. A formulary is a list of prescription drugs covered by a prescription drug plan. Also known as a drug list, it's usually broken down into tiers. Tier 1 drugs are likely to be covered more comprehensively than those in tiers 2 and 3.

in-network. In-network providers have a contract with the health insurance company in which they've agreed to certain terms, including specific costs. Your expenses will usually be less with in-network providers and the process may be simpler.

out-of-network. Out-of-network providers don't have a contract with the health insurance company related to how care is covered or specific costs of care. Seeing out-of-network providers may mean paying higher out-of-pocket expenses or having no coverage at all.

out-of-pocket expenses. Out-of-pocket expenses are the expenses you pay after your insurance company has covered all it's going to pay. Most policies have an annual out-of-pocket maximum. This means there's a limit to the amount you have to pay out of your own pocket in a year.

outsourcing. This is the practice in which a treatment facility refers you to a health care provider who's not part of their program. This can affect your costs since the outsourced providers may not be in-network.

GENERAL INFORMATION

The federal Mental Health Parity and Addiction Equity Act (MHPAEA) of 2009 requires insurance companies to treat and cover mental health disorders in the same manner as any other health-related problem. The act states that health insurance plans cannot have higher copays and other out-of-pocket expenses for behavioral health claims than for other medical claims. How this act is applied varies by state.

Many treatment programs accept insurance or government payment in the form of:
- State-financed health insurance.
- Medicaid.
- Medicare.
- Private insurance.
- Company-covered services.

Be aware that health insurance providers are not required to cover costs of treatment related to relapses. If you relapse, you may need to pay for the treatment yourself.

Most health insurance companies have websites that include information for policyholders, including lists of in-network and out-of-network providers, coverage information and steps in the process. This website is listed on your insurance card.

If you don't find the website helpful or if you prefer to talk to someone in person, call the customer service number on the back of your insurance card. Allow a significant amount of time to make these calls and be prepared to be placed on hold for quite a while.

WHERE TO START

If you feel that all of this is more than you can handle, consider asking someone to help you make phone calls and gather information.

Make sure to record the names of all people you speak to, contact numbers, and dates and times you talked. You may need to make several calls and it can be hard to remember all the details, so keep notes.

It's generally best to call the treatment program first so you know what questions you need to ask your insurance company. The program you're considering may have a website that includes information regarding questions you have.

After you have spoken with the treatment program and have the information you need, then call the insurance company.

Questions for the treatment program you are considering

Key questions include:
- Will staff members arrange insurance preauthorization for you? If yes, is it for all services or only some?

- Are any of the treatment services outsourced? If yes, which ones?

Questions for the insurance company

When talking with your insurance company, these are some of the terms you may need to reference to determine your coverage:
- Addiction treatment services.
- Mental health services.
- Substance abuse disorder services.
- Drug and alcohol rehabilitation programs.

Questions about general coverage

- What services are covered under my plan?
- What services require preauthorization?
- Do I need a physician's referral for treatment to receive coverage?
- Is the program or provider I am considering in-network?
- If the program outsources some of my treatment to out-of-network providers, how are those costs covered?
- Does coverage vary depending on whether the treatment is inpatient or outpatient?
- How many days of treatment are covered? How many treatments are covered?
- Does my policy cover costs related to relapse?
- Is there any other information I should know?

Questions about copays, deductibles and out-of-pocket expenses

- Do I have a deductible? If yes, how much is it and have I met it yet?
- What is my copay?
- Do my copays vary depending on the service?
- What is my annual out-of-pocket maximum?

Questions about medications

- How are medications for opioid use disorder (MOUD) covered?
- How can I access your list of approved medications (formulary)?
- How can I determine the cost of medications?

IF YOU DON'T HAVE INSURANCE

Unfortunately, not everyone has health insurance. Even those who do have insurance may not have enough coverage to afford care. In addition, if an insurance company decides that a certain service isn't medically necessary, that service may not be covered. This is true even if the service is important to your recovery process.

If you don't have insurance or if you need help with expenses, contact a social services agency in your community or a community-based health care center that's government funded. State-sponsored health care coverage typically covers addiction treatment services.

CHANGING POLICY COVERAGE

When you talk to your insurance company, you may decide that you want to make changes to your coverage before you receive treatment. If you're the policy owner, you can make changes to the policy. If someone else is the policy owner, that person has to make the changes.

How to give naloxone

IMMEDIATELY follow these steps if you suspect someone is overdosing from an opioid:

1. Call 911 or emergency medical help.
2. Check your surroundings to ensure you are safe. Look for traffic, needles, loose powder or other dangers.
3. Follow the directions given to you by the 911 or emergency medical help operator. This may include giving the person CPR if you are comfortable doing so.
4. Give naloxone using one of the methods listed here.

I overdosed in my family's house. My family was all there. All I remember is my family trying to wake me up. They called 911. Thankfully, the paramedics worked fast. They gave me naloxone twice. They did CPR. When I came to, I was on the floor and a paramedic said, "You just died."

This was very traumatic for my family. It was traumatic for me knowing I was seconds away from being dead on my grandpa's birthday.

_____

CHEYENNE,
25 YEARS OLD

GIVING NALOXONE USING THE READY-TO-USE NASAL SPRAY (NARCAN)

1. Lay the person on their back.

2. Open the naloxone package.

3. Tilt the person's head back. Put your hand under the person's neck to provide support.

4. Place your index and middle finger on the sides of the nozzle. Place your thumb on the bottom.

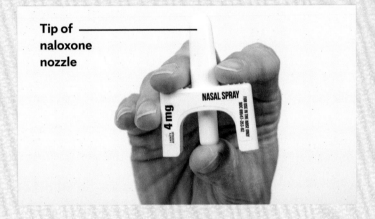

Tip of naloxone nozzle

5. Insert the tip of the nozzle into one nostril until your fingers touch the person's nose.

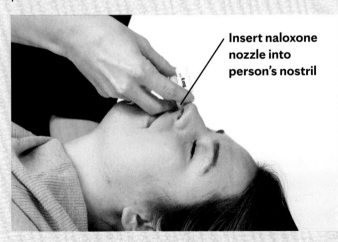

Insert naloxone nozzle into person's nostril

6. Use your thumb to push the bottom firmly to deliver the naloxone.

7. Keep the person's airway clear by rolling the person onto their side. Position the person's hands under their head. Position the knee to keep the person from rolling onto their stomach. If the person vomits, this position can help prevent the person from choking.

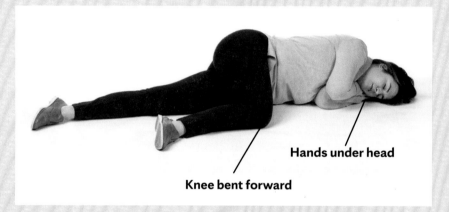

Hands under head

Knee bent forward

8. If the person doesn't begin to breathe within three minutes, give another dose if you have one. Follow the 911 or emergency medical help operator's directions about whether to try giving CPR again.

9. If the person doesn't respond or breathes and then stops breathing again, give another dose with a new nasal spray if you have one.

10. When the emergency team arrives, give them as much information as you can, including the number of times you gave naloxone and the person's response to it.

GIVING NALOXONE USING THE PREFILLED SYRINGE WITH A NASAL ATOMIZER

An atomizer is a device that turns fluid into a mist. It has a white foam tip that you attach to the top of the plastic tube. The atomizer fits in the person's nostril.

1. Lay the person on their back.

2. Open the packages and take out the contents.

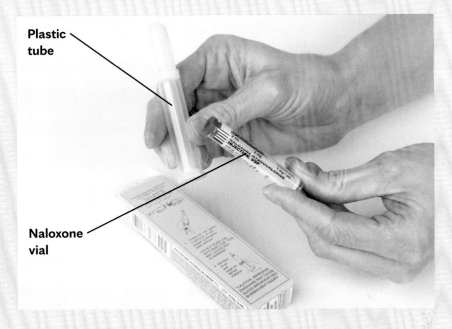

Plastic tube

Naloxone vial

3. Locate the white foam tip.

4. Remove the caps from the top and bottom of the plastic tube.

5. Remove the cap from the top of the naloxone vial.

6. Gently attach the white foam tip to the top of the plastic tube.

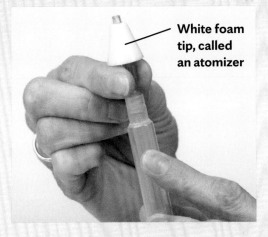

White foam tip, called an atomizer

7. Gently thread — don't push — the naloxone vial into the plastic tube by twisting it about three-and-a-half turns. Make sure the needle within the plastic tube has pierced the rubber stopper at the top of the naloxone vial.

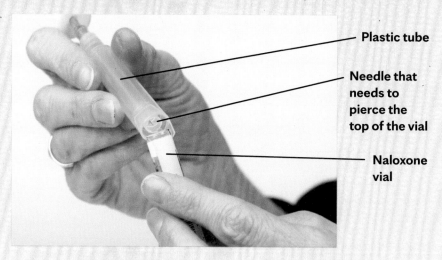

Plastic tube

Needle that needs to pierce the top of the vial

Naloxone vial

8. Tilt the person's head back.

9. Insert the white foam tip into one nostril. Give a firm push on the end of the naloxone vial to give half the naloxone into one nostril. Then insert the white foam tip into the other nostril and give the other half of the naloxone.

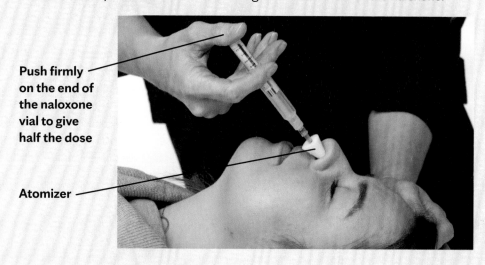

Push firmly on the end of the naloxone vial to give half the dose

Atomizer

10. Keep the person's airway clear by rolling the person to the side. Position the person's hands under their head. Position the knee to keep the person from rolling onto their stomach. If the person vomits, this position can help prevent the person from choking

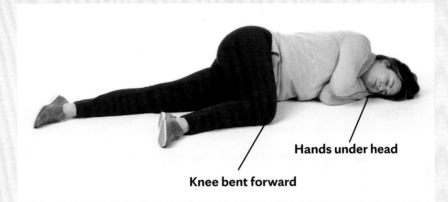

Hands under head

Knee bent forward

11. If the person doesn't begin to breathe within three minutes, give another dose if you have one. Follow the 911 or emergency medical help operator's directions about whether to try giving CPR again.

12. If the person begins to breathe and then stops breathing again, give another dose with a new naloxone vial, if you have one.

13. When the emergency team arrives, tell them as much information as you can, including the time you gave the naloxone and the person's response to it.

GIVING NALOXONE BY INJECTING IT INTO A MUSCLE

1. Lay the person on their back or side so that you can easily get to the person's arm or leg.

2. Open the package and take out the contents.

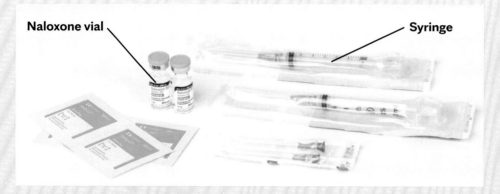

3. Remove the plastic cap from the top of the naloxone vial. Use an alcohol swab to wipe the top of the naloxone vial three times.

4. Remove the syringe from the package. Remove the plastic cap at the top of the syringe that covers the needle.

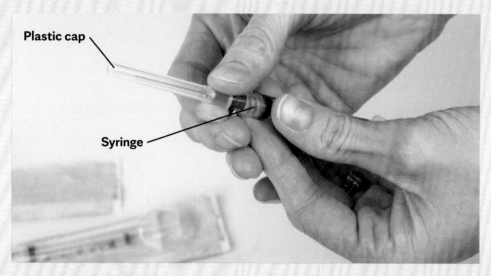

5. Push the needle into the rubber top of the naloxone vial.

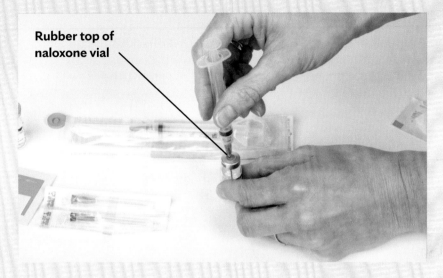

Rubber top of naloxone vial

6. Tip the bottle upside down. Make sure the tip of the needle is in the naloxone solution. Pull back on the plunger of the syringe to draw up 1 mL of naloxone. The syringe has measurement lines on it. Make sure there's only naloxone in the syringe and no air. If there's air, push on the plunger gently until only a very small amount of naloxone comes out of the needle tip.

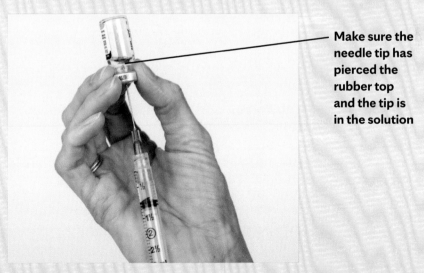

Make sure the needle tip has pierced the rubber top and the tip is in the solution

7. Use an alcohol wipe to swab the injection site. Inject the naloxone into a big muscle, such as the person's outer thigh or upper arm.

8. Keep the person's airway clear by rolling them to the side. Position the person's hands under their head. Position the knee to keep the person from rolling onto their stomach. If the person vomits, this position can help prevent them from choking.

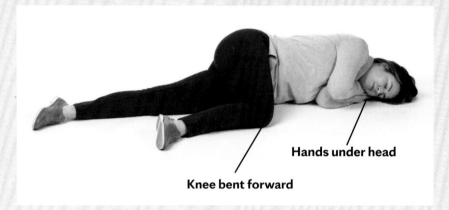

Hands under head

Knee bent forward

9. If the person doesn't begin to breathe within three minutes, give another dose if you have one. Follow the 911 or emergency medical help operator's directions about whether to try giving CPR again.

10. If the person begins to breathe and then stops breathing again, give another dose if you have one.

11. When the emergency team arrives, tell them as much information as you can, including the time you gave the naloxone and the person's response to it.

Index

M